ICSA Book Series in Statistics

Series Editor

Ding-Geng Chen, College of Health Solutions
Arizona State University
Chapel Hill, NC, USA

The ICSA Book Series in Statistics showcases research from the International Chinese Statistical Association that has an international reach. It publishes books in statistical theory, applications, and statistical education. All books are associated with the ICSA or are authored by invited contributors. Books may be monographs, edited volumes, textbooks and proceedings.

Jeffrey R. Wilson • Kent A. Lorenz
Lori P. Selby

Modeling Binary Correlated Responses

Using SAS, SPSS, R and STATA

Second Edition

Springer

Jeffrey R. Wilson
Arizona State University
Department of Economics, W.P. Carey
School of Business
Tempe, AZ, USA

Kent A. Lorenz
Department of Kinesiology
San Francisco State University
San Francisco, CA, USA

Lori P. Selby
Arizona State University, School of
Mathematics and Statistics
Tempe, AZ, USA

ISSN 2199-0980 ISSN 2199-0999 (electronic)
ICSA Book Series in Statistics
ISBN 978-3-031-62426-1 ISBN 978-3-031-62427-8 (eBook)
https://doi.org/10.1007/978-3-031-62427-8

This Springer imprint is published by the registered company Springer Nature Switzerland AG
The registered company address is: Gewerbestrasse 11, 6330 Cham, Switzerland

This book is dedicated to my grandson Willem Wilson-Ellis, my three daughters, Rochelle, Roxanne, and Rhonda, and all my statistics students past and present at Arizona State University.

Jeffrey R. Wilson

My parents, Rose and Arnold, and all my family and friends.

Kent A. Lorenz

My parents Patricia Selby, Urick Selby, mentors Joseph L. and Teresa Abraham, my family and friends.

Lori P. Selby

Preface

The main focus of this book is on the modeling of binary response data. Binary outcomes can be observed directly or through the dichotomization of a continuous variable; however, binary data analysis has some unique challenges when compared to continuous data analysis. Some potential issues a researcher needs to consider when analyzing binary data are as follows:

- Are the trials based on a mechanism that produces independent or correlated observations?
- Are the data based on repeated measures or are they cross-sectional?
- Are the covariates time dependent or time independent?
- Are the covariates entered into the model as a fixed or random effect?
- Are there marginal models being fitted or subject-specific models? In other words, is the interest to model the mean or to be subject specific?

This book is based on real examples and data we have encountered over several years of research and teaching statistics at the Master's and PhD levels at Arizona State University. In fact, several of the chapters are based on the applied projects and theses of Master's and PhD students in the university's statistics programs. The examples in this book are analyzed whenever possible using SAS, SPSS, R, and STATA. While the SAS, SPSS, R, and STATA outputs are contained in the text with partial data tables, the completed datasets can be found at the web address https://www.public.asu.edu/~jeffreyw.

The aim of this book is to concentrate on making complicated ideas and propositions comprehendible, specifically those ideas related to modeling different types of binary response data (Fig. 1). The chapters in this book are designed to help guide researchers, practitioners, and students (at the senior or Master's degree levels who have some basic experience with regression as well as some knowledge of statistical packages like SAS, SPSS, R, and STATA) in understanding binary regression models using a variety of application areas.

This book presents existing studies and recent developments in statistical methods, focusing on their applications to correlated binary data and other related research. The data and computer programs used throughout the text and analyzed

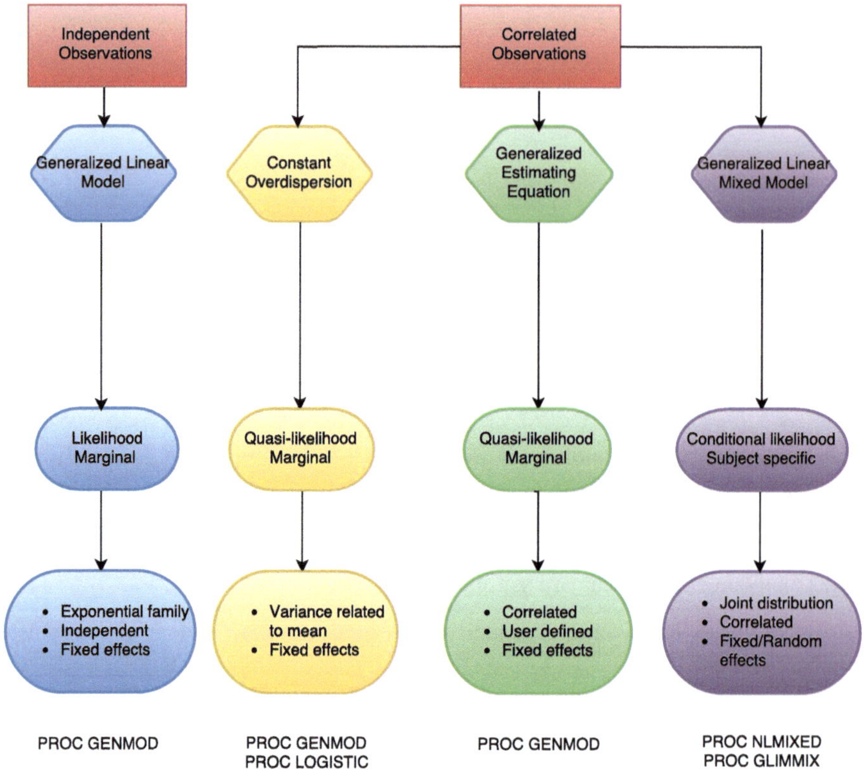

Fig. 1 Types of binary models

using SAS, SPSS, R, and STATA are publicly available so that readers can replicate the models and the results presented in each chapter. This allows the reader to easily apply the data and methods to his or her own research. The book strives to bring together in one place the key methods used in the analysis of dependent observations with binary outcomes, and presents and discusses recent issues in statistical methodological development, as well as their applications. The book is timely and has the potential to impact model development and correlated binary data analyses of health and health-related research, education, banking, and social studies, among others. In an academic setting, the book could serve as a reference guide for a course on binary data with overdispersion, particularly for students at the graduate level (master's or doctoral students) seeking degrees in related quantitative fields of study, though not necessarily in statistics. In addition, this book could serve as a reference for researchers and data analysts in education, the social sciences, public health, and biomedical research.

Each chapter consists of seven sections and is organized as follows:

Section 1: Motivating Example

1.1 Description of the Case Study
1.2 Study Hypotheses

Section 2: Definitions and Notations
Section 3: Exploratory Analyses
Section 4: Statistical Model
Section 5: Analysis of Data
Section 6: Conclusions
Section 7: Examples

The book comprises five major parts, and all of the chapters are arranged within them. Below, we provide a short summary for each of the chapters found within the four major parts of the book.

Part I: Introduction and Review of Modeling Uncorrelated Observations

1. Introduction to Binary Logistic Regression
   Statistical inference with binary data presents many challenges, whether or not the observations are dependent or independent. Studies involving dependent observations tend to be longitudinal or clustered in nature and, therefore, provide inefficient estimates if the correlation in the data is ignored. This chapter, then, reviews binary data under the assumption that the observations are independent. It provides an overview of the issues to be addressed in the book, as well as the different types of binary correlated data. It introduces SAS, SPSS, R, and STATA as the statistical programs used to analyze the data throughout the book and concludes with general recommendations.
2. Short History of the Logistic Regression Model
   The logistic regression model, as compared to the probit, Tobit, log–log, and complementary log–log models, is worth revisiting based upon the work of Cramer (2002, 2003). The ability to model the odds has made the logistic regression model a popular method of statistical analysis, in addition to the fact that the model can be used for prospective, retrospective, or cross-sectional data while the probit, Tobit, log–log, and the complementary log–log models can only be used with prospective data to model probability. This chapter provides a summary of Cramer's work (2002, 2003) and relies heavily on Cramer's own excellent but terse history of the evolution of the logistic regression model.
3. Standard Binary Logistic Regression Model
   The logistic regression model is a type of predictive model that can be used when the response variable is binary, as in the cases of: live/die, disease/no disease, purchase/no purchase, win/lose, etc. In short, we want to model the probability of getting a certain outcome by modeling the mean of the variable (which

is the same as the probability in the case of binary variables). A logistic regression model can be applied to response variables with more than two categories; however, those cases, though mentioned in this text, are less common. This chapter also addresses the fact that the logistic regression model is more effective and accurate when analyzing binary data as opposed to the simple linear regression. We will therefore present three significant problems that a researcher may encounter if the linear regression model was fitted to binary data:

1. There are no limits on the values predicted by a linear regression, so the predicted response (mean) might be less than 0 or greater than 1, which is clearly outside the realm of possible values for a response probability.
2. The variance for each subpopulation is different and therefore not constant. Since the variance of a binary response is a function of the mean, if the mean changes from subpopulation to subpopulation, the variance will also change.
3. Usually, the response is binary and so the assumption of normal distribution is not appropriate in these cases.

The chapter provides an example using cross-sectional data and a binary (two-level) response, and then fits the model in SAS, SPSS, R, and STATA. The models are based on data collected for one observation per sampling unit, and the chapter also summarizes the application to independent binary outcomes. There are several excellent texts on this topic, including Agresti (2002), which is referenced in the chapter.

Part II: Analyzing Correlated Data Through Random Component

4. Overdispersed Logistic Regression Model

   When binary data are obtained through simple random sampling, the covariance of the responses follows the binomial model (two possible outcomes from independent observations with constant probability). However, when the data are obtained under other circumstances, the covariances of the responses differ substantially from the binomial case. For example, clustering effects or subject effects in repeated measure experiments can cause the variance of the observed proportions to be much larger than the variances observed under the binomial assumption. The phenomenon is generally referred to as overdispersion or extra variation. The presence of overdispersion can affect the standard errors and, therefore, also affect the conclusions made about the significance of the predictors. This chapter presents a method of analysis based on work presented in:

   Wilson, J. R., & Koehler, K. J. (1991). Hierarchical models for cross-classified overdispersed multinomial data. *Journal of Business and Economic Statistics*, *9*(1), 103–110.

5. Weighted Logistic Regression Model

Binary responses, which are common in surveys, can be modeled through binary models that can provide a relationship between the probability of a response and a set of covariates. However, as explained in Chap. 4, when the data are not obtained by simple random sampling, the standard logistic regression is not valid. Rao and Scott (1984) show that when the data come from a complex survey designed with stratification, clustering, and/or unequal weighting, the usual estimates are not appropriate. In these cases, specialized techniques must be applied in order to produce the appropriate estimates and standard errors. Clustered data are frequently encountered in fields such as health services, public health, epidemiology, and education research. Data may consist of patients clustered within primary care practices or hospitals, or households clustered within neighborhoods, or students clustered within schools. Subjects nested within the same cluster often exhibit a greater degree of similarity, or homogeneity of outcomes, compared to randomly selected subjects from different clusters (Austin et al., 2001; Goldstein, 1995; Kreft & De Leeuw, 1998; Raudenbush & Bryk, 2002; Snijders & Boskers, 1999). Due to the possible lack of independence of subjects within the same cluster, traditional statistical methods may not be appropriate for the analysis of clustered data. While Chap. 4 uses the overdispersed logistic regression and the exchangeability logistic regression model to fit correlated data, this chapter incorporates a series of weights or design effects to account for the correlation. The logistic regression model on the analysis of survey data takes into account the properties of the survey sample design, including stratification, clustering, and unequal weighting. The chapter fits this model in SAS, SPSS, and R, using methods based on:

Koehler, K. J., & Wilson, J. R. (1986). Chi-square tests for comparing vectors of proportions for several cluster samples. *Communications in Statistics*, *15* (10), 2977–2990.
Wilson, J. R. (1986). Approximate distribution and test of fit for the clustering effect in Dirichlet multinomial model. *Communications in Statistics*, *15*(4), 1235–1249.
Wilson, J. R. (1989). Chi-square tests for overdispersion with multiparameter estimates. *Journal of Royal Statistics Society Series C, Applied Statistics*, *38*(3), 441–454.

6. Generalized Estimating Equation Logistic Regression Model

Many fields of study use longitudinal datasets, which usually consist of repeated measurements of a response variable, often accompanied by a set of covariates for each of the subjects/units. However, longitudinal datasets are problematic because they inherently show correlation due to a subject's repeated set of measurements. For example, one might expect a correlation to exist when looking at a patient's health status over time or a student's performance over time. But in those cases, when the responses are correlated, we cannot readily obtain the underlying joint distribution; hence, there is no closed-form joint likelihood function to present, as with the standard logistic regression model. One remedy is to fit a generalized estimating equations (GEE) logistic regression model for the data, which is explored in this chapter. This chapter addresses repeated measures of the sampling unit, showing how the GEE method allows missing values within a subject without losing all the data from the subject, and time-varying predictors that can appear in the model. The method requires a large number of subjects and provides estimates of the marginal model parameters. We fit this model in SAS, SPSS, R, and STATA, basing our work on the method best presented by Ziang and Leger (1986), and Liang and Zeger (1986).

7. Generalized Method of Moments Logistic Regression Model

   When analyzing longitudinal binary data, it is essential to account for both the correlation inherent from the repeated measures of the responses and the correlation realized because of the feedback created between the responses at a particular time and the covariates at other times (Fig. 2). Ignoring any of these correlations can lead to invalid conclusions. Such is the case when the covariates are time dependent and the standard logistic regression model is used. Figure 2 describes two types of correlations: responses with responses and responses with covariates. We need a model that addresses both types of relationships. In Fig. 2, the different types of correlation presented are as follows:

   1. There is the correlation among the responses which are denoted by $y_1, \ldots, y_T$ as time t goes from 1 to T.
   2. There is the correlation between response Y_t and covariate X_s:
      (a) When responses at time t impact the covariates in time $t + s$
      (b) When the covariates in time t impact the responses in time $t + s$

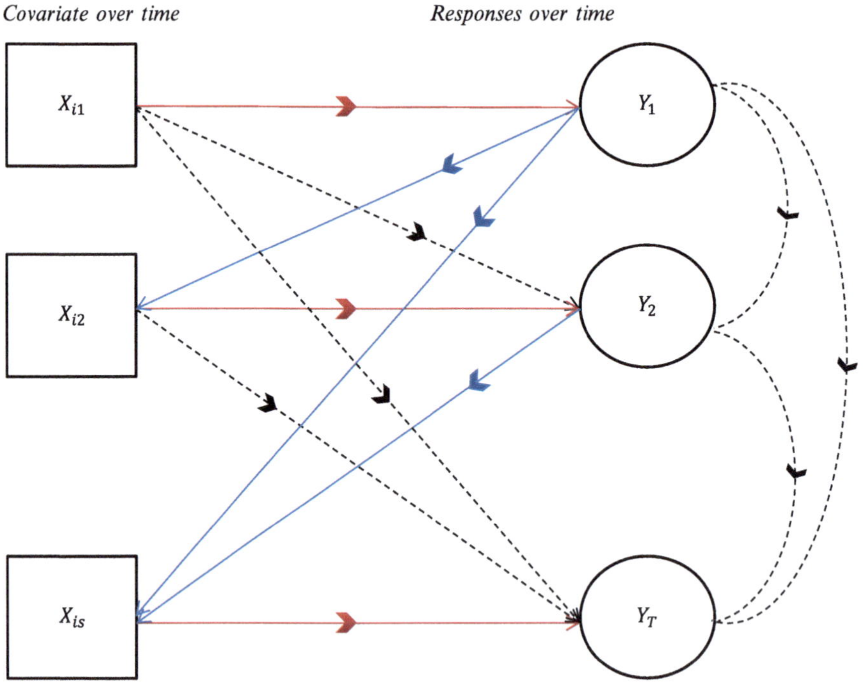

Fig. 2 Two types of correlation structures

These correlations regarding feedback from Y_t to the future X_{t+s} and vice versa are important in obtaining the estimates of the regression coefficients.

This chapter provides a means of modeling repeated responses with time-dependent and time-independent covariates. The coefficients are obtained using the generalized method of moments (GMM). We fit these data with SAS Macro (Cai & Wilson, 2015) using methods based on:

LaLonde, T., Wilson, J. R., & Yin, J. (2014). GMM logistic regression models for longitudinal data with time-dependent covariates and extended classifications. *Statistics in Medicine*, *33*(27).

8. Exact Logistic Regression Model

   As computers' abilities to do tedious calculations have increased, using exact logistic regression models has become more popular in healthcare, banking, and other industries. Traditional methods (which are based on asymptotic theory) when used for analyzing small, skewed, or sparse datasets are not usually reliable. When sample sizes are small or the data are sparse or skewed, exact conditional inference is necessary and applicable (Derr, 2008). Exact methods of inferences are based on enumerating the exact distributions of certain statistics to estimate the parameters of interest in a logistic regression model, conditional on the remaining parameters. This is a method of testing and estimation that uses conditional methods to obtain exact tests of parameters in binary and nominal logistic models. Exact methods are appropriate for small-sample or sparse data situations that often result in the failure (nonconvergence or separation) of the usual unconditional maximum likelihood estimation method. However, exact methods can take a great deal of time and memory as sample or model sizes increase. For sample sizes too large for the default exact method, a Monte Carlo method is provided. The chapter uses EXACT statement in PROC LOGISTIC or PROC GENMOD, and we also fit models in SAS, C+, and R. Our methods are based on:

   Troxler, S., Lalonde, T. L., & Wilson, J. R. (2011). Exact logistic models for nested binary data. *Statistics in Medicine*, *30*(8).

Part III: Analyzing Correlated Data Through Systematic Components

9. Two-Level Nested Logistic Regression Model

   Studies including repeated measures are expected to give rise to correlated data. Such data are common in many disciplines including healthcare, banking, poll tracking, and education. Subjects or units are followed over time and are repeatedly observed under different experimental conditions, or are observed in clusters. Often times, such data are available in hierarchical structures consisting of a subset of a population of units at several levels. We review methods that include the clustering directly in the model (systematic component) as opposed to methods that include the clustering within the random component. These methods belong to the class of generalized linear mixed models. The basic idea behind generalized linear mixed models is conceptually straightforward (McCulloch, 2003) and incorporates random effects into the systematic component of a generalized linear model to account for the correlation. Such approaches are most useful when researchers wish to account for both fixed and random effects in the model. The desire to address the random effects in a logistic model makes it a subject-specific model. This is a conditional model that can also be used to model longitudinal or repeated measures data. We fit this model in SAS, SPSS, and R. Our method of modeling is based on:

Lalonde, T., Nguyen, A. Q., Yin, J., Irimata, K., & Wilson, J. R. (2013). Modeling correlated binary outcomes with time-dependent covariates. *Journal of Data Science, 11*(4), 715–738

10. Hierarchical Logistic Regression Model
    This chapter expands upon the results of Chap. 9. It is common to come into contact with data that have a hierarchical or clustered structure. Examples include patients within a hospital, students within a class, factories within an industry, or families within a neighborhood. In such cases, there is variability between the clusters, as well as variability between the units, which are nested within the clusters. Hierarchical models take into account the variability at each level of the hierarchy and thus allow for the cluster effects at different levels to be analyzed within the models (Shahian et al., 2001). This chapter tells how one can use the information from different levels to produce a subject-specific model. We concentrate on fitting logistic regression models to these kinds of nested data at three levels and higher (Fig. 3). In Fig. 3, as an example, patients are nested within doctors and doctors are nested within hospitals. This is a three-level nested design but can be expanded to higher levels, though readily available computing may be challenge.
11. Fixed Effects Logistic Regression Model
    If a researcher wants to know whether having a job reduces recidivism among chronic offenders, that researcher could compare an individual's arrest rate when he/she is employed with his/her arrest rate when unemployed.

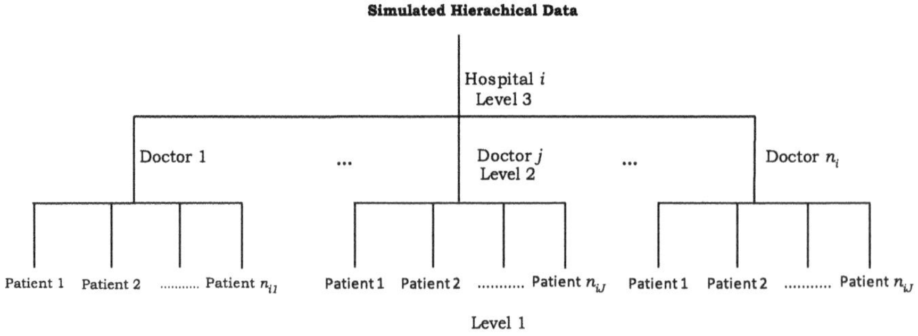

Fig. 3 Hierarchical structure of three levels

The difference in arrest rates between the two periods is an estimate of the employment effect for that individual. Similarly, a researcher might want to know how a child's performance in school differs depending on how much time he/she spends watching television. The researcher could compare how the child does when spending significant time watching television versus when he/she does not watch television. Fixed effects logistic regression models can be used for both of these scenarios. Such models are used to analyze longitudinal data with repeated measures on both the response and the covariates. These models treat each measurement on each subject as a separate observation, and the set of subject coefficients that would appear in an unconditional model are eliminated by conditional methods. This is a conditional, subject- specific model (as opposed to a population-averaged model like the GEE model). We fit this model in SAS, SPSS, and R. An excellent discussion with examples can be found in P. D. Allison (2005), *Fixed Effects Regression Methods for Longitudinal Data Using SAS*. For binary response data, we use the STRATA statement in PROC LOGISTIC.

Part IV: Analyzing Correlated Data Through the Joint Modeling of Mean and Variance

12. Heteroscedastic Logistic Regression Model

    Correlated binomial data can be modeled using a mean model if the interest is only on the mean and the dispersion is considered a nuisance parameter. However, if the intraclass correlation is of interest, then there is a need to apply a joint modeling of the mean and the dispersion. Efron (1986) was one of the first to model both the mean and the variance. The dispersion sub-model allows extra parameters to model the variance independent of the mean, thus allowing covariates to be included in both the mean and variance sub-models. In this chapter, we present a sub-model that analyzes the mean and a sub-model that analyzes the variance. This model allows both the dispersion and the mean to be modeled. We use the MODEL statement in the SAS/ETS procedure QLIM to specify the model for the mean and use the HETERO statement to specify the dispersion model. We fit this model in SAS and SPSS. Our results and presentation are based on work done in some recent masters' research papers at Arizona State University.

Part V: Case Studies: USA Election 2020 and Netherlands COVID

13. Case Studies: Analysis of Election Data and Covid Data

    We take a practitioner view of 2020 Election Data in the United States of America and address certain questions with views to the 2024 election. We also did a similar approach to COVID data as they data were collected over time.

The authors of this book owe a great deal of gratitude to many who helped in the completion of the book. We have been fortunate enough to work with a number of graduate students at Arizona State University: Anh Nguyen, who provided the graphics and had a lot to do with extracting and analyzing the Medicare dataset in the initial stages; Hong Xiang, who, through her master's applied paper, contributed to findings regarding PROC NLMIXED and hierarchical analyses; Jianqiong Yin, who provided insight and unwavering contributions to our statistical programming through her thesis and associated work; Katherine Cai, who helped with SAS Macro; and Chad Mehalechko, who provided overwhelming support in doing the SAS, SPSS, and R programming for all chapters. Many thanks to the staff in the Department of Economics and the computing support group in the W. P. Carey School of Business. To everyone involved in the making of this book, we say thank you!

Finally, a special thanks to our families, who have provided us with the support needed to achieve this great endeavor.

Tempe, AZ, USA — Jeffrey R. Wilson
San Francisco, CA, USA — Kent A. Lorenz
Tempe, AZ, USA — Lori P. Selby

Contents

Part III Analyzing Correlated Data Through Systematic Components

Part I
Introduction and Review of Modeling Uncorrelated Observations

Chapter 1
Introduction to Binary Logistic Regression

1.1 Motivating Example

The need to profile or describe a unit/subject based on a binary outcome is often of utmost importance. While there are other models (e.g., probit, log-log, complementary log-log) that can be used to model binary responses, in this book, we concentrate on logistic regression models. The advantage of the logistic regression model lies in the model's ability to explain and predict the outcomes in terms of the odds and how applicable it is to cases where the data are obtained from prospective, retrospective, or cross-sectional settings. For example, we wish to detect the factors which determine whether patient's cancer is in remission. In that simulated study data, there is a three-level hierarchical structure with patients nested within doctors within hospitals. The study is part of a large study of lung cancer outcomes across multiple doctors and sites. The response variable is whether or not the cancer is in remission. The covariates at the patient level are age, length of stay, family history, and cancer stage. At the doctor's level, we have their identification and their years of experience. At the hospital level, we have the hospital identification.

This book deals with the topic of logistic regression models concentrating on binary data. The statement leads naturally to the following questions:

- What is a binary logistic regression model?
- What do we mean by binary data?
- Why do we need logistic regression models?
- Why is it not adequate to use the standard regression analysis to analyze binary data?

J. R. Wilson et al., *Modeling Binary Correlated Responses*, ICSA Book Series in Statistics, https://doi.org/10.1007/978-3-031-62427-8_1

1.2 Definition and Notation

1.2.1 Notation

Let N denote the number of units in the population, while n denotes the sample size, and T times $t = 1, \ldots T$; with J covariates $j = 1, \ldots J$.

1.2.2 Definitions

A *variable* is defined as any measure that varies from unit to unit (i.e., individual to individual or subject to subject). For example, if we measured the blood pressure for 10 individuals, we would expect the values to be different, making blood pressure the "variable" of interest. Another example of a variable would be measuring the ages of 8000 Japanese-American men to analyze the variable of age.

The *output* variable Y is also called the *response* variable, or *dependent* variable or *outcome* variable or *target* variable. It is the variable of interest.

A *quantitative* variable is an individual measure taken on a numerical scale. It is often referred to as a continuous variable, meaning that these observations may lie on a continuum. Thus, a *continuous* variable takes on an infinite number of possible values, and its reported value is limited only by physical measurement accuracy. We will make references to quantitative variables measured on two scales as follows:

An *interval scale* pertains to variables that can be ordered and give precise measures of the distances between categories. Measuring temperature in degrees Celsius is an example of this type of quantitative variable.

A *ratio scale* is for ratio variables, which are interval variables with a true zero value. Using temperature as our example, a reading of zero degrees on the Celsius scale does not actually denote an absence of heat or energy. Therefore, we classify it as an interval variable. However, zero degrees on the Kelvin scale refer to an absolute zero, or an absence of temperature or energy. Therefore, we classify it as a ratio variable. A key difference between interval and ratio scales is that, with ratio scales, the distance between measurements may be equal (i.e., the difference between 10 °C and 20 °C is the same as between 25 °C and 35 °C. However, 20 °C is not twice as much "temperature" as 10 °C. Only when using a ratio scale could you make those statements (i.e., 20 K is twice as much as 10 K)).

A *qualitative* variable is one whose values vary in type rather than in magnitude. It expresses a qualitative attribute, meaning that its values are not numerical. The observations cannot be said to vary in magnitude, and a natural hierarchical ordering is not possible.

A binary random variable is usually symbolized or coded as a 1 or 0. It is appropriate when the assessment of a characteristic is in terms of any two categories such as yes/no, present/absent, and favorable/unfavorable. These are called categories. The corresponding variable is called *binary* or *dichotomous* or *indicator*. The coded values do not have any meaning or rank, so they cannot be interpreted numerically. However, several statistical programs require one or zero coding for analysis. With a zero or one coded value, a researcher can find the mean. Such a summary value is referred to as the proportion. Examples include: "Do you smoke?" Proportion: those who smoke. Or "Do you drink?" Proportion: those who drink. Thus, the mean of a binary variable is called the proportion.

A *categorical* variable is a variable measured on a nominal scale whose categories determine class or group membership. A *categorical* variable can take "values" which denote nonnumerical categories or classes. Some definitions are: A *categorical* variable represents a set of discrete events, such as groups, decisions, or anything else that can be classified into categories. Categorical variables are also referred to as discrete variables, meaning a limited set of numerical values that are typically counting numbers or whole numbers. Two main types of categorical variables are nominal and ordinal variables.

Ordinal variable consists of a rank, or a rating. One example would be: "How was the performance?" Some possible responses on a measurement scale could be: 1 for "Excellent," 2 for "Above Average," 3 for "Average," 4 for "Below Average," and 5 for "Poor." There is an obvious limitation to this type of measurement: The examiner cannot be assured of the preciseness of a measurement like satisfaction. In this example, "Excellent" is higher than "Above Average," but it is not very precise because it does not show how much higher an "Excellent" rating is compared to an "Above Average" rating. This limitation also means that there can be no guarantee that a difference between a score of 1 and 2 is the same as a difference between a score of 4 and 5.

Nominal variable has characteristics that are mutually exclusive and exhaustive. This means that nominal variables can only be measured in terms of whether an individual belongs to a certain category. Some examples are: "What region of the country are you from (Northeast, Northwest, Midwest, etc.)?" or "Are you single, married, widowed, or divorced?"

Categorical Variable in the Form of a Series of Binary Variables

Categorical variables can be reformulated and treated like a set of binary variables.

Consider the categorical variable "Region," with levels (East, West, North, and South).

When converted to four binary variables representing "Region," it looks like the following:

1. East with levels (yes, no)
2. West with levels (yes, no)
3. North with levels (yes, no)
4. South with levels (yes, no)

Example: Consider the following data given about "Region" in Table 1.1.

Table 1.1 Dichotomization of a categorical variable

Observations	Region	East	West	North	South
#124	East	1	0	0	0
#246	South	0	0	0	1
#513	North	0	0	1	0
#734	West	0	1	0	0

Instead of the variable called "Region," we now have East, West, North, and South. Thus, the focus will be on binary and continuous variables. However, when we reformulate a categorical variable into a series of binary variables, we use all but one to represent the categorical variable going forward. In our example, we can use East, West, and North as binary variables to represent *Region* for any modeling. Information about South is achieved by letting East, West, and North take on a value of 0 instead of 1. When interpreting the binary variable coefficient and significance, it is compared to the one category that is left out.

Relationship Between Response and Predictor Variables

The *response variable* is the variable of interest to the experimenter. The main goal of an experiment usually is to determine if there are some relationships between the predictor variable and the response variable. There are two types of relationships that are used to explain the relationship between the predictor variables and the response variable: "functional" or "statistical." When a relationship can be expressed by a mathematical formula or expression, then this is known as a *functional relationship*. For example, Distance = Velocity by Time. The other type of relationship is called a *statistical relationship*.

A statistical relationship is not exact and has two identifiable markers: First, an experimenter knows there is a statistical relationship when the response variable has a distribution associated with it (known or unknown) and has a relationship that can be described by the mean and its predictor variables in a systematic fashion. This relationship would give rise to a line (one predictor) or plane (two or more predictors) with the expected value as the central point of a distribution of possible responses. In addition, with statistical relationships there will be a variation of the Y observations around the systematic part. For example, the relationship between blood pressure after an experiment and blood pressure before an experiment would be a statistical relationship (Fig. 1.1).

1.3 Exploratory Analyses

Consider the following diagram, Fig. 1.2. This is our input-output system where X is the input and Y is the output. Figure 1.2 provides a diagrammatic view of a set of predictors (binary, continuous, or categorical) being fed into a system from which a

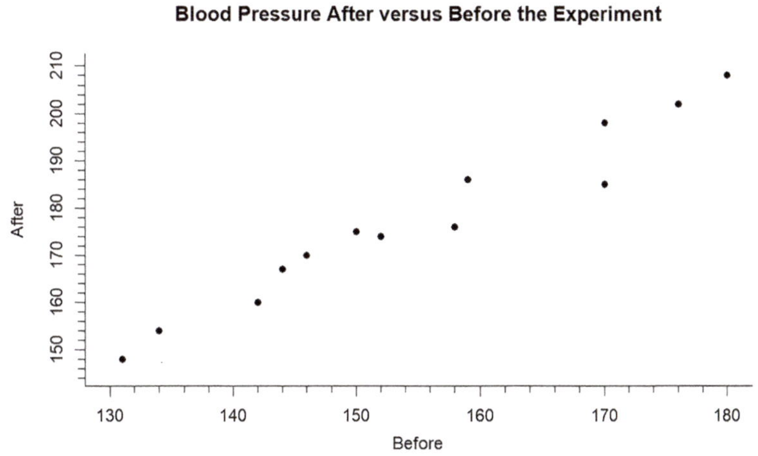

Fig. 1.1 Two-dimensional graph

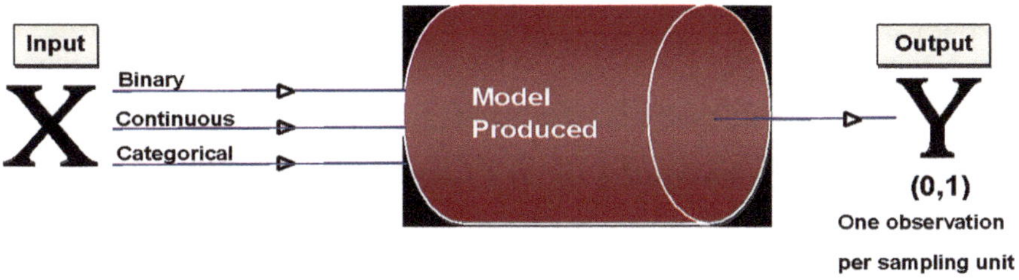

Fig. 1.2 An input-output system

binary output is produced. Each production relies on a single sampling unit independent of other units.

In Fig. 1.2, *Y* denotes the output variable in the system, and *X* represents the set of input variables also referred to as independent, explanatory, concomitant, prognostic factor, predictor, driver, covariate, or factor variables, depending on the discipline. Our known information denoted by *X* can be any combination of quantitative or binary variable or categorical variable, while Y can be one of quantitative, binary, or categorical. We will concentrate on binary response in Y.

A general view of most statistical models is that we have a set of covariates with known information, being placed into a system that produces a known outcome. We refer to such as the input variable(s) and the outcome produced, the output variable. The set of variables going into or coming out of the system may be of different kinds:

- *Quantitative:* like age in years, income, or weight
- *Binary:* like gender, smoker, or eligible to vote
- *Categorical:* like race, region, or marital status

The output variable produced from this system can be binary, quantitative, or categorical, but in this chapter, we focus on binary responses.

1.4 Statistical Models

Logistic or logit regression models are very common in the fields of healthcare, business, banking, and sociology. We categorize these models into the following:

- Single response versus repeated responses on the sampling unit
- Population-averaged versus subject-specific model
- Fixed versus random effects
- Time-independent versus time-dependent covariates
- Responses as binary

This book provides an overview of modeling binary responses through logistic regression models. Though we do mention nominal and ordinal models, we concentrate mainly on binary response cases. We investigate independent versus correlated responses, cross-sectional versus longitudinal data, time-dependent versus time-independent covariates, fixed versus random effects, and subject-specific versus population-averaged models. We fit most of these types of models using either SAS, SPSS, R, or STATA.

This book covers the following topics and statistical models:

1.4.1 Chapter 3: Standard Binary Logistic Regression Model

We use a binary (two-level) response and examine cross-sectional data. We fit this model in SAS, SPSS, R, and STATA. We present models based on data collected for one observation per sampling unit where the observations are considered to be independent.

1.4.2 Chapter 4: Overdispersed Logistic Regression Model

When binary data are not obtained through simple random sampling, the covariance for the sample proportion can differ substantially from the covariance corresponding to the binomial model. We present a model based on a factor for the correction of the overdispersion. We fit this model in S SAS, SPSS, R, and STATA.

1.4.3 Chapter 5: Survey Data Logistic Regression Model

The logistic regression model on the analysis of survey data incorporates properties of the survey sample design, including stratification, clustering, and unequal weighting. We fit this model in SAS, SPSS, and R.

1.4.4 Chapter 6: Generalized Estimating Equations (GEE) Logistic Regression Model

This chapter addresses repeated measures on the sampling unit. The generalized Estimating Equations (GEE) method allows missing values within a subject without losing all the data from the subject, and time-dependent predictors can appear in the model. The method requires a large number of subjects and provides estimates of the marginal or population-averaged model parameters. We fit this model in SAS, SPSS, R, and STATA.

1.4.5 Chapter 7: Generalized Method of Moments (GMM) Logistic Regression Model

This model provides a means of modeling repeated responses with time-dependent and time-independent covariates. The coefficients are obtained using generalized method of moments. We fit these data with PROC IML in SAS.

1.4.6 Chapter 8: Exact Logistic Regression Model

This is a method of testing and estimation that uses conditional methods to obtain exact tests of parameters in binary and nominal logistic models. We found that asymptotic methods are not appropriate for small sample sizes or sparse data situations because they often result in failure (nonconvergence or separation) if the usual unconditional maximum likelihood estimation method is used. However, exact methods can take a great deal of time and memory as the sample size or number of parameters increases. We use the EXACT statement in PROC LOGISTIC or PROC GENMOD. We fit models in SAS, C+, and R.

1.4.7 Chapter 9: Two-Level Nested Logistic Regression Model

It allows random effects in a logistic model, resulting in a subject-specific model. This is a conditional model that can also be used to model longitudinal or repeated measures data. We use PROC GLIMMIX, but the model can also be fitted in PROC NLMIXED by using a different methodology that typically limits the number of random effects to one or two. However, in recent research, we show how it can be expanded. We fit this model in SAS, SPSS, R, and STATA.

1.4.8 Chapter 10: Hierarchical Logistic Regression Model

These models are applicable for cases where responses are taken more than once on each unit (or item), either at multiple times or under multiple conditions. There are three primary types of models: marginal (or population-averaged), subject-specific (includes fixed effects and random-effects model), and transitional. We use the NLMIXED procedure to fit models and concentrate on the subject-specific models. We fit these models in SAS and R.

1.4.9 Chapter 11: Fixed Effects Logistic Regression Model

This model treats each measurement on each subject as a separate observation, and the set of subject coefficients that would appear in an unconditional model are eliminated by conditional methods. This is a conditional, subject-specific model (as opposed to a population-averaged model like the GEE model). We fit this model in SAS, SPSS, R, and STATA.

1.4.10 Chapter 12: Heteroscedastic Logistic Regression Model

The heteroscedastic logistic regression model allows the dispersion and mean to be modeled. We use the MODEL statement in the procedure QLIM to specify the model for the mean and use the HETERO statement to specify the dispersion sub model. We fit this model in SAS.

1.4.11 Chapter 13: Case Studies—Election Data and COVID Data

The election data provide a combined sample of the MIT Election Data and Science Lab about the 2020 US presidential election by state and county (https://dataverse.harvard.edu/dataset.xhtml?persistentId=doi:10.7910/DVN/42MVDX) with data from the US Census Bureau. Our aim is to predict the successful candidate based upon socioeconomic factors of the region from poverty estimates for US States (2021) data (U.S. Department of Commerce, Bureau of the Census, Small Area Income and Poverty Estimates (SAIPE) Program: https://www.census.gov/programs-surveys/saipe.html).

Election Data Analysis

1. **Hypothesis:** Socioeconomic factors, such as poverty rates, educational attainment, and income levels, are predictive of the successful candidate in the 2020 US presidential election at the state and county level.
   - Analysis: Build logistic regression models to investigate the association between socioeconomic variables (e.g., poverty estimates) and the likelihood of voting for a particular candidate (e.g., Republican or Democrat) in each state and county.
2. **Hypothesis:** Demographic factors, such as racial composition and urban/rural divide, play a significant role in determining the outcome of the 2020 US presidential election.
   - Analysis: Incorporate demographic variables from the US Census Bureau into logistic regression models to examine their impact on the probability of voting for a specific candidate.
3. **Hypothesis:** There are regional variations in the relationship between socioeconomic factors and voting behavior, reflecting differing political landscapes and priorities across states and counties.
   - Analysis: Explore interactions between socioeconomic variables and geographical regions (states, counties) in logistic regression models to identify differential effects on voting outcomes.

We use some models introduced in this book to analyze hypotheses as they relate to COVID *data* and to *election data*. The COVID data analysis was due to an article by Dr. Marc Jacobs (https://medium.com/@marc.jacobs012/predicting-covid-19-mortality-using-logistic-regression-in-sas-5453d3532cd7). It reports on data from provinces in the Netherlands about the probabilities of hospitalizations and mortality due to COVID-19 across a 1-year span (Data source: https://data.rivm.nl/covid-19/).

COVID-19 Data Analysis

1. **Hypothesis:** Socioeconomic factors, such as poverty levels and access to healthcare, impact the probabilities of COVID-19 hospitalizations and mortality in different provinces of the Netherlands.
   - Analysis: Conduct logistic regression modeling to assess the relationship between socioeconomic variables (e.g., poverty rates) and COVID-19 outcomes (hospitalizations and mortality) across provinces.
2. **Hypothesis:** There are temporal trends in COVID-19 mortality and hospitalization probabilities over the 1-year span covered by the data.
   - Analysis: Examine how the probabilities of COVID-19 hospitalizations and mortality change over time within each province using logistic regression with time-series data.

3. **Hypothesis:** The effectiveness of public health interventions (e.g., lockdown measures, vaccination campaigns) varies across provinces and is associated with differences in COVID-19 outcomes.
   - Analysis: Evaluate the impact of public health interventions on COVID-19 mortality and hospitalization probabilities using logistic regression while controlling for other relevant factors.

1.5 Analysis of Data

Throughout this book, we fit several types of the logistic regression models, as previously mentioned. These models can consist of one or more of the following:

- Independent or correlated responses
- Covariates that change with time and/or those that do not
- Fixed and/or random effects
- Marginal or subject-specific

Figure 1.3 summarizes the content of each chapter in the book. In each chapter, we describe the model and then provide an analysis of a dataset based on a particular model using SAS, SPSS, R, and STATA, whenever possible.

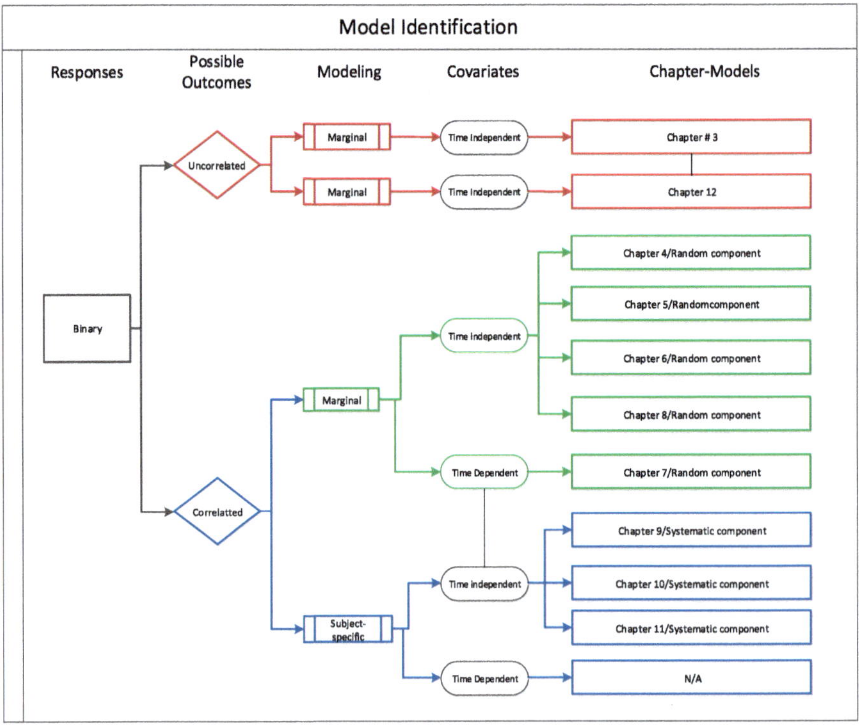

Fig. 1.3 Chart of binary models

1.5.1 SAS Programming

SAS is a programming language that has powerful capabilities for data manipulation, statistical analysis, report writing, and generating plots. SAS was developed in the early 1970s at North Carolina State University and stands for "Statistical Analysis System." The Institute was founded in 1976 by two North Carolina State University professors, Dr. James Goodnight and Dr. John Sall. The two professors developed a statistical analysis software package that became popular with faculty at a number of universities first throughout the South and expanded into the rest of the country. Because of its capabilities and popularity, we will use SAS programming for much of the modeling in this book.

1.5.2 SPSS Programming

SPSS (Statistical Package for the Social Sciences) is a data management and analysis program produced by SPSS, Inc., Chicago. First created in 1968, it is a software package used for conducting statistical analyses, manipulating data, and generating tables and graphs that summarize data. Statistical analyses range from basic descriptive statistics, such as averages and frequencies, to advanced inferential statistics, such as regression models, analysis of variance, and factor analysis. SPSS has several capabilities for manipulating data, recoding data, and computing new variables, including merging and aggregating datasets. SPSS, like SAS, can summarize and display data in the form of tables and graphs.

1.5.3 R Programming

R is an implementation of the S language, a language for manipulating objects. R provides a suite of software facilities for statistically analyzing data, manipulating data, as well as computing and displaying the results. R is a programming environment for data analysis and graphics. The book *S Programming* by Venables and Ripley (2000) provides a comprehensive overview of programming principles using S and R. For more details on the S language, readers are referred to Becker et al. (1988) and Venables and Ripley (2002). It is our understanding that the language was initially written by Ross Ihaka and Robert Gentleman at the Department of Statistics at the University of Auckland. Since then, many analysts and researchers have contributed to the package. R provides a platform for the development and implementation of new algorithms and technology transfer. One can use R in three possible ways: using functions that make use of existing algorithms within R, using functions that call on external programs written in either C or FORTRAN, or combining pieces of code that have specific parts attached to handle certain aspects of the data.

1.5.4 STATA Programming

STATA is a full-featured statistical package similar to SAS and SPSS. There are different versions of STATA, but each version provides a complete set of manuals in PDF format, hyperlinked to the online help. STATA differs in some other packages in requiring that the entire dataset to be analyzed must reside in memory. STATA runs the same way on Windows, Mac OS X, Unix, and Linux systems. STATA has three major strengths: data manipulation, statistics, and graphics. STATA is an excellent tool for data manipulation:

- Moving data from external sources into the program
- Cleaning it up
- Generating new variables
- Generating summary datasets
- Merging datasets and checking for merge errors
- Collapsing cross–section time-series data on either of its dimensions
- Reshaping datasets from "long" to "wide" and so on.

As such, STATA is an excellent program for answering questions about any aspect of the data. STATA provides the standard univariate, bivariate, and multivariate statistical tools, from descriptive statistics and t-tests through one-way ANOVA, two-way ANOVA, and multi-way ANOVA, regression, principal components. It has a very powerful set of techniques for the analysis of limited dependent variables: logit, probit, ordered logit and probit, multinomial logit, and other binary models.

1.5.5 Fitting Models

We fit most of these models using SAS, SPSS, R,and STATA procedures, though at times we may only use SAS. We have the book organized based on the responses (independent or correlated) and the assumptions of correlation, if correlated then part of random component or part of systematic component.

- We begin with one measurement per sampling unit and model the mean.
  - When the data originate from an independent source
  - When the data are overdispersed
  - When the data are from surveys

- We look at cases when more than one response comes from the sampling unit.
  - When the responses are correlated
  - When the responses are correlated but the data are hierarchical
- We look at cases with repeated measures and time-dependent covariates.
- We look at cases with fixed effects.
- We look at exact methods.
- We look at joint modeling of mean and dispersion.

1.6 Conclusions

Even though we have been studying techniques for analyzing logistic regression data since the early 1980s, we are still impressed by the continual need for more methods to analyze binary data. We have used logistic regression models to find construction defects, model FDA submissions, analyze heart surgery data, profile shoplifters, conduct *High School and Beyond* data analyses, model statistics for patient rehospitalization, identify cheating on the LSAT, and more. We know that there are many papers on the topic of logistic regression models. However, we wanted to make sure that non-statisticians could have a full understanding of the applications of logistic regression models without needing a rigorous, in-depth education on the topic. We wrote this book to serve that purpose.

A binary logistic regression model can be used to identify the predictors that influence the binary outcome. Binary data is the result of one of two possible outcomes. The logistic regression is necessary since we must be certain that predicted values lie between [0, 1]. Also, the usual regression has a mean that is not related to the variance. It is not sufficient to use the usual regression analysis. The usual regression satisfies the assumptions required for continuous data. The fitting of logistic regression models is widespread and readily accepted across several disciplines. Each chapter in this book addresses the fit of binary logistic regression models under varying conditions. We begin each chapter with questions that readers may be interested in as they analyze the datasets. We hope that the way we present the material makes it easy for you to use SAS, SPSS, R, and STATA to analyze your data.

1.7 Related Examples

Our data examples are used by graduate students at Arizona State University in theses and applied projects in their pursuit of a graduate degree in statistics. We describe the datasets as they will be used in the chapters throughout the text. These data are available at www.public.asu.edu/~jeffreyw.

1.7.1 Medicare Data

Medicare is a social insurance program administered by the US government, providing health insurance coverage to people who are aged 65 and over or who meet other special criteria. Medicare currently pays for all rehospitalization, except those in which patients are rehospitalized within 24 h after discharge for the same condition for which they had initially been hospitalized (Jencks et al., 2009). We extracted data from the Arizona State Inpatient Database (SID) for use in this textbook. Our dataset contains patient information from Arizona hospital discharges for a 3-year period from 2003 through 2005. This dataset contains information for those who are admitted to a hospital exactly four times. We selected diseases based on the seven most common diseases and three procedures that accounted for 50% of hospitalizations in Arizona hospitals for the period 2003–2005. There are 1626 patients in the dataset with complete information; each has three observations indicating three different instances of rehospitalization.

1.7.2 Philippines Data

Data were collected by the International Food Policy Research Institute in Bukidnon Province in the Philippines and focused on quantifying the association between body mass index (BMI) and morbidity 4 months into the future. Data are collected at four time points, separated by 4-month intervals (Bhargava, 1994). There are 370 children with 3 observations on each child. The predictors are BMI, age, gender, and time as a categorical variable, but represented by two indicator variables.

1.7.3 Household Satisfaction Survey

Brier (1980) examined data from a study of housing satisfaction performed by H. S. Stoeckler and M. G. Gate for the US Department of Agriculture. Households around Montevideo, Minnesota, are stratified into two populations: those in the metropolitan area and those outside the metropolitan area. A random sample of 20 neighborhoods is taken from each population, and 5 households are randomly selected from each of the sampled neighborhoods. One response is obtained from the residents of each household concerning their satisfaction with their home. The possible responses are "unsatisfied" (US), "satisfied" (S), and "very satisfied" (VS). Only data from neighborhoods in which responses are obtained from each of the five households sampled are used to illustrate the usefulness of the model. This reduces the original dataset to $K_1 = 18$ neighborhoods from the nonmetropolitan area and $K_2 = 17$ neighborhoods from the metropolitan area. These data are analyzed using a Dirichlet multinomial model (Koehler & Wilson, 1986).

1.7.4 NHANES: Treatment for Osteoporosis

This example uses the *demoadv* dataset, a subset from the National Health and Nutrition Examination Survey (NHANES) database (Centers for Disease Control and Prevention, 2009). We want to know the association between calcium supplement use (*anycalsup*) and the likelihood of receiving treatment for osteoporosis (*treatosteo*) among participants, aged 20 years and older, after controlling for selected covariates. The covariates include gender (*riagendr*), age (*ridageyr*), race/ethnicity (*ridreth1*), and body mass index (*bmxbmi*). Information on the use of vitamin, mineral, herbal, and other dietary supplements is collected from all NHANES participants during the household interview.

Stage 1: Primary sampling units (PSUs) are selected from strata defined by geography and proportions of minority populations. These are mostly single counties or, in a few cases, groups of contiguous counties selected with probability proportional to a measure of size (PPS). Most strata contain two PSUs. Additional stages of sampling are performed to select various types of secondary sampling units (SSUs), namely, the segments, households, and individuals that are selected in Stages 2, 3, and 4.

Stage 2: The PSUs are divided into segments (generally city blocks or their equivalent). As with each PSU, sample segments are selected with PPS.

Stage 3: Households within each segment are listed, and a sample is randomly drawn. In geographic areas where the proportion of age, ethnic, or income groups selected for over-sampling is high, the probability of selection for those groups is greater than in other areas.

Stage 4: Individuals are chosen to participate in NHANES from a list of all persons residing in selected households. Individuals are drawn at random within designated age-sex-race/ethnicity screening sub-domains. On average, 1.6 persons are selected per household.

1.7.5 COVID Data

Data source: https://data.rivm.nl/covid-19/. The analysis of hospitalizations and mortality due to COVID-19 based upon province, gender, and age group across a 1-year span from data from the Netherlands. The analysis is due Dr. Marc Jacobs (https://medium.com/@marc.jacobs012/predicting-covid-19-mortality-using-logistic-regression-in-sas-5453d3532cd7) and includes adjustments to clustering and overdispersion.

1.7.6 Election Data

To help explore hierarchical analysis, we combined data from the MIT Election Data and Science Lab about the 2020 US presidential election by state and county with data from the US Census Bureau on county-level socioeconomic factors. From the presidential election data spreadsheet, we selected 12 states that were matched for location and population (6 states voted for the Democratic candidate [Arizona, California, Georgia, Illinois, New York, and Pennsylvania], and 6 voted for the Republican candidate [Florida, Indiana, Ohio, Texas, South Carolina, Utah]). Votes for each candidate by state and county were summed and compared using Microsoft Excel for Windows to produce a binary outcome variable (0 = Democratic candidate won state/county; 1 = Republican candidate won state/county). There are two levels of data present: by state as a whole and by county within state.

https://dataverse.harvard.edu/dataset.xhtml?persistentId=doi:10.7910/DVN/42MVDX

In order to predict the successful candidate based upon socioeconomic factors of the region, we combined the presidential winner by county data with data from poverty estimates for US States (2021) data available from the US Department of Commerce, Bureau of the Census, Small Area Income and Poverty Estimates (SAIPE) Program (https://www.census.gov/programs-surveys/saipe.html). The data were organized by state and county, and we selected the following predictor variables:

- Rural-Urban Continuum Code, 2013
- Estimate of people of all ages in poverty 2021
- Estimated percent of people of all ages in poverty 2021
- Estimate of related children aged 5–17 in families in poverty 2021
- Estimated percent of related children aged 5–17 in families in poverty 2021
- Estimate of median household income 2021

References

Becker, R. A., Chambers, J. M., & Wilks, A. R. (1988). *The new S language*. Wadsworth & Brooks.

Bhargava, A. (1994). Modelling the health of Filipino children. *Journal of the Royal Statistical Society. Series A (Statistics in Society), 157*, 417–432.

Brier, S. S. (1980). Analysis of Contingency Tables Under Cluster Sampling. *Biometrika, 67*(3), 591–596. https://doi.org/10.2307/2335128

Centers for Disease Control and Prevention (CDC). (2009). National Center for Health Statistics (NCHS). National Health and Nutrition Examination Survey Data. Hyattsville, MD: U.S. Department of Health and Human Services, Centers for Disease Control and Prevention.

Jencks, S. F., Williams, M. V., & Coleman, E. A. (2009). Rehospitalizations among patients in the Medicare fee-for-service program. *New England Journal of Medicine, 360*(14), 1418–1428.

Koehler, K. J., & Wilson, J. R. (1986). Chi-square tests for comparing vectors of proportions for several cluster samples. *Communications in Statistics - Theory and Methods, 15*, 2977–2990.

Venables, W., & Ripley, B. D. (2000). *S programming*. Springer.

Venables, W., & Ripley, B. D. (2002). *Modern Applied Statistics* (4th ed.). ISBN 0-387-95457-0.

Chapter 2
Short History of the Logistic Regression Model

2.1 Motivating Example

More than 175 years after the advent of the growth curve, we have fully embraced the logistic regression model as a viable tool for binary data. Today, the logistic regression model is one of the most widely used binary models in the analysis of categorical data. The logistic regression model is based on modeling the odds of an outcome, and the idea of odds (as used commonly by the researcher) has lots of appeal. Many researchers seem to be familiar with the odds of certain outcomes, whether their discussions are on sports, illness, or almost anything else. Additionally, it is quite interesting from a statistical point of view that whether the data were obtained from prospective design, retrospective design, or cross-sectional design, the covariate's impact on the binary outcome will be the same.

Since this book concentrates on fitting logistic regression models, it is reasonable to spend a little time rehashing the history and the origination of binary models. The advent of the logistic regression model, as compared to the probit, Tobit, log-log, and complementary log-log models, is worth revisiting (Cramer, 2002, 2003). The ability to model the odds has made it very attractive since the logistic regression relies on the odds, and the odds can always be computed whether the data are prospective design, a retrospective design, or a cross-sectional. However, since the probit, Tobit, log-log, and complementary log-log models rely on probabilities, they are only applicable to prospective data. Logistic regression models model the probability (nonlinear) or, equivalently, the odds (nonlinear) or logit (linear) of the outcome of an event. Logistic regression models have been used in countless ways, analyzing anything from election data to credit card data to healthcare data. Logistic regression analysis is a useful tool for these disciplines because it is ideal for identifying, discriminating, and profiling different types of subpopulations.

J. R. Wilson et al., *Modeling Binary Correlated Responses*, ICSA Book Series in Statistics, https://doi.org/10.1007/978-3-031-62427-8_2

2.2 Definition and Notation

2.2.1 Notation

In this discussion, we use the following symbols:

P_t is the probability of the outcome at time t being one.
$1 - P_t$ is the probability of the outcome being zero at time t.
log is the natural logarithm.
logit denotes the log of the odds, i.e., (log $[P_t/(1 - P_t)]$.
β_0 represents the value of the logit when the covariate is zero.
β_1 represents the increase in the logit for a unit increase in the covariate (when continuous) or the difference from one category to the next if the covariate is binary.

2.2.2 Definition

A monotonic function is a function which is either entirely nonincreasing or nondecreasing. A function is said to be monotonic if its rate of increase or decrease remains the same in direction. So for $x > 0$ then $f(x) = x^2$ is monotonic increasing since $f(x + 2) > f(x)$ for any $x > 0$ but is not for all x.

A probit model is a type of regression for binary data on a scale that depends on the cumulative distribution function of normal distribution.

A prospective study is a study designed to determine the relationship between an outcome and certain characteristic of the units involved. The researcher follows the population group over a period of time, noting the event or nonevent (e.g., lung cancer) occurs in the smokers and in the nonsmokers. Prospective studies produce an opportunity to determine probabilities for each group (event or nonevent) and as such provide the relative risk.

A retrospective study **is** a study in which the event or nonevent is unknown and the information gathered depends on what occurred in the past. One example is a study of patients with AIDS and whether or not they had used dirty needles or other common practices.

A case-control study is a nonexperimental research design. We collect information on previous cases and compare with a control group of persons who have not had that case (called the control). The two groups (case and control) are matched for age, sex, and other personal data and are examined to determine which possible factor (e.g., cigarette smoking, watched television) may account for the increase or decrease in the case group.

A Tobit model also called a censored regression model is suitable for linear relationships between variables when there is either left- or right-censoring in the dependent variable. Example: In the 1980s, there was a federal law restricting speedometer readings to no more than 85 mph. So, if you wanted to try and predict a vehicle's top speed from a combination of horsepower and engine size, you would get a reading no higher than 85, regardless of how fast the vehicle was really traveling. This is a classic case of right-censoring (censoring from above) of the data. The one thing we are certain about is that those vehicles recorded as traveling at 85 mph were at least 85 mph. Introduction to SAS. UCLA: Statistical Consulting Group. http://www.ats.ucla.edu/stat/sas/notes2/ (accessed November 24, 2007).

2.3 Exploratory Analyses

The logistic regression model is a tool for presenting the relation between a binary response or a multinomial response and several predictors. Its use is very familiar and common in the fields of health and education, as well as with elections, credit card companies, mortgage, and other cases, where there is need to profile the sampling unit (Fig. 2.1).

Some example questions to guide a study might be as follows:

1. How do education, ideology, race, and gender predict a vote in favor or not in favor of a US senator?
2. What factors predict the type of registered voters who would support the reelection of a president or governor?
3. What are the characteristics of the consumer who should be offered a credit card?
4. What characteristic of the traveler will make him or her choose one mode of transportation over another (rail, bus, car, or plane)?

2.4 Statistical Model

The origin of the logistic regression model has its roots in bioassay besides some other disciplines. One report tells us that the logistic function was invented to describe population growth and given its name by a Belgian mathematician named Verhulst. Figure 2.2 provides a description of the function:

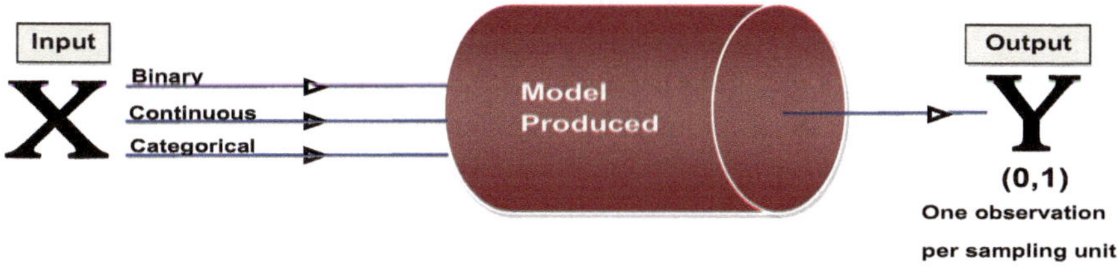

Fig. 2.1 A schematic diagram as X impacts Y

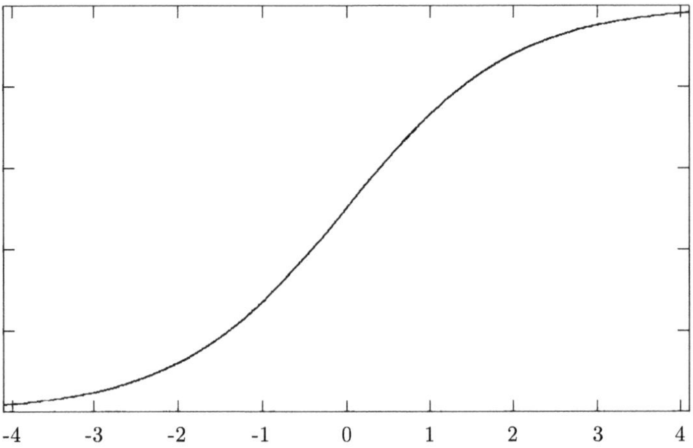

Fig. 2.2 A logistic curve P_t versus time

$$P_t = e^{\beta_0 + \beta_1 t} / \left[1 + e^{\beta_0 + \beta_1 t}\right]$$

This figure shows the relation of proportion P_t as time increases. Let the linear relation be

$$\text{logit}\left[P_t\right] = \beta_0 + \beta_1 t,$$

where β_0 denotes the value at time equal to zero, β_1 denotes the rate of change of logit $[P_t]$ with regards to time, and

$$\text{logit}\left[P_t\right] = \log\left[P_t / \left(1 - P_t\right)\right]$$

The logistic function rises monotonically as t increases. We concur with authors who have noted that for P_t from 0.3 to 0.7, the shape of the logistic curve closely resembles the normal probability cumulative distribution function (Fig. 2.3).

One account of the emergence of the use of the logistic function from the growth curve dated as far back as 1838 as it became a popular formula for certain places in North Africa (Cramer (2002)). In more recent times, Dr. Pearl of the US Food Administration was preoccupied with the food needs of a growing population during World War I and decided to use logistic functions to address it. Additionally, President Dr. Lowell Reed of Johns Hopkins used an application of the logistic curve to catalysis caused by a catalytic agent formed during a reaction (Reed & Berkson, 1929). The logistic function was also used in chemistry at the same time, but it appears that the basic idea was for logistic growth. This is still used to this day to model population growth and market penetration of new products and technologies.

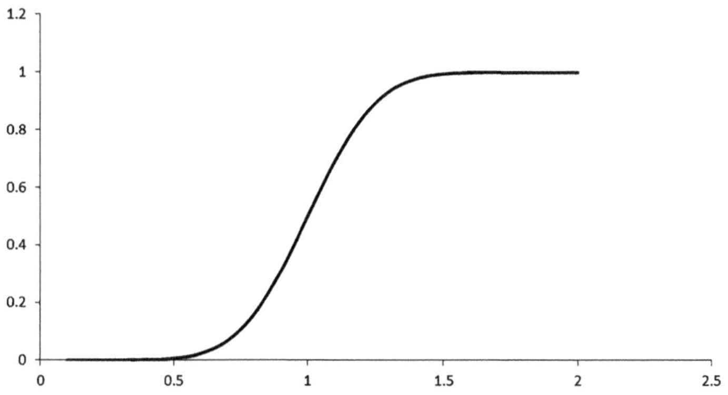

Fig. 2.3 Cumulative distribution function of normal distribution

There is a close resemblance of the logistic to the normal distribution function (Wilson (1925) and Winsor (1932). As an alternative to normal probability function *in* 1944, Berkson turned his attention to the statistical methodology of bioassay and proposed the use of the logistic instead of the normal probability function of P_t, coining the term "logit" by analogy to the "probit" as presented by Cramer. The logit model of bioassay is easily generalized to logistic regression where binary outcomes are related to a number of determinants, without a specific theoretical background.

We learned that the earliest developments in statistics and epidemiology took place in the late 1950s and the 1960s. We learned in the discipline of statistics that the analytical advantages of the logit transformation as a means of dealing with discrete binary outcomes were at the forefront. This was supported by Dr. Cox as a pioneer in the field by publishing a series of papers in the 1960s about the topic and then following them up with the outstanding textbook titled *Analysis of Binary Data* (Cox, 1969). Later, the close proximity of the logistic model with discriminant analysis was recognized, as well as its unique relationship to log linear models (Bishop et al., 1975). We further learned that epidemiologists were busy developing case-control studies even earlier, and since these are directly concerned with odds, and odds ratios, the log-odds or logit transformation arises naturally. It appears that researchers were already clamoring about the theoretical justification (Cornfield, 1951, 1956), and we must mention the works of Berkson (1944, 1951).

Our research led us to believe that the first comprehensive textbook with medical applications was published by Hosmer and Lemeshow (1989). I remember using their first edition in my graduate categorical data class in statistics at Arizona State University shortly after I arrived in Tempe. Until recently, I was unaware that I was touching part of history. I remember back then talking to some researchers from the marketing department and being told that logistic regression was brought to their discipline by certain researchers. The presence of logistic regression models in behavioral sciences is believed to be to the works of McKelvey and Zavoina.

They adopted the approach based on an ordered probit analysis of the voting behavior of US congressmen. However, the generalization of logistic regression to the multinomial or polychotomous case was due to Gurland et al. (1960), Cox (1969), Mantel (1966), and Theil (1969).

2.5 Analysis of Data

Our analyses of binary data with logistic regression models will be done mostly with SAS, SPSS, and R. There are several procedures in SAS, SPSS, R, and STATA for modeling binary responses under varying conditions and certain assumptions. We attempt to use the most common procedures as we demonstrate the fit of logistic regression models to correlated data with and without time dependent covariates and with fixed and random effects. There are a few chapters when we were unable to duplicate the fit of the model in all three statistical packages.

2.6 Conclusions

The logistic regression is often preferred as a model for binary responses as it is appropriate for any kind of data: cross-sectional, prospective, and retrospective. Its reliance on the odds makes it an excellent candidate for interpretation as society can easily relate to such. On the other hand, probit or complementary log-log is only appropriate for modeling prospective data as they rely on probabilities.

References

Berkson, J. (1944). Applications of the logistic function to bioassay. *Journal of the American Statistical Association, 9*, 357–365.

Berkson, J. (1951). Why I prefer logits to probits. *Biometrics, 7*(4), 327–339.

Bishop, Y. M., Fienberg, S. E., & Holland, P. W. (1975). *Discrete multivariate analysis: Theory and practice*. MIT Press.

Cornfield, J. (1951). A method of estimating comparative rates from clinical data. *Journal of the National Cancer Institute, 11*, 1269–1275.

Cornfield, J. (1956). A statistical problem arising from retrospective studies. In J. Neyman (Ed.), *Proceedings of the third Berkeley symposium on mathematical statistics and probability* (pp. 135–148). University of California Press.

Cox, D. R. (1969). *Analysis of binary data*. Chapman and Hall.

Cramer, J. S. (2002). *The origins of logistic regression*. Tinbergen Institute Working Paper No. 2002–119/4. Available at SSRN: http://ssrn.com/abstract=360300 or https://doi.org/10.2139/ssrn.360300

Cramer, J. S. (2003). The origins and development of the logit model. In *Logit models from economics and other fields* (pp. 149–158).

Gurland, J., Lee, I., & Dahm, P. A. (1960). Polychotomous quantal response in biological assay. *Biometrics, 16*, 382–398.

Hosmer, D., & Lemeshow, W. (1989). *Applied logistic regression*. Wiley.

Mantel, N. (1966). Models for complex contingency tables and polychotomous response curves. *Biometrics, 22*, 83–110.

Reed, L. J., & Berkson, J. (1929). The application of the logistic function to experimental data. *Journal of Physical Chemistry, 33*, 760.

Theil, H. (1969). A multinomial extension of the linear logit model. *International Economic Review, 10*(3), 251–259.

Wilson, E. B. (1925). The logistic or autocatalytic grid. *Proceedings of the National Academy of Science, 11*, 431–456.

Winsor, C. P. (1932). A comparison of certain symmetrical growth curves. *Proceeding of Washington Academy of Science, 22*, 73–84.

Chapter 3
Standard Binary Logistic Regression Model

The chapter provides an example using cross-sectional data and a binary (two-level) response while fitting the model in SAS, SPSS, R, and STATA. The models are based on data collected for one observation per sampling unit, and the chapter also summarizes the application to independent binary outcomes. There are several excellent texts on this topic, including Agresti (2002), which is referenced in this chapter.

3.1 Motivating Example

Hospital administrators were convinced they could predict rehospitalization within 30 days of a patient's release based on the number of procedures each patient had undergone, the length of stay, and the number of diseases connected with each patient at the time of dismissal. They collected a random selected set of charts for 1625 patients to see if they could predict future outcomes based on that sample of data. In the collected data, the response variable is binary (rehospitalized in 30 days versus not), so the use of a multiple linear regression model, which is appropriate with continuous response variable, would not be appropriate.

3.1.1 Study Hypotheses

The administrators wanted to know if the number of procedures, length of stay, and number of diseases associated with each patient were significant predictors of rehospitalization. They were particularly interested in knowing how they could predict the rehospitalization of future patients based on these characteristics. In a sense, they wanted to be able to profile the patients, a practice that is not unique to

J. R. Wilson et al., *Modeling Binary Correlated Responses*, ICSA Book Series in Statistics, https://doi.org/10.1007/978-3-031-62427-8_3

rehospitalization research. Profiling is common in other scenarios such as admissions processes for colleges and universities where administrators use predictors to determine whether a prospective student will be successful in their programs.

3.2 Definition and Notation

Sampling unit is the item or subject exposed to the measurement of the response independently of other units. It constitutes a single value for the variable of interest. It may consist of a single element, or groups of elements.

Subpopulation is a set of units belonging to a distinct combination of the covariate values in the data.

Proportion is the mean of a binary variable and referred to as the probability. It stems from coding your outcomes as 1 or 0 and finding the average.

Sampling error describes the variation among identically and independently treated sampling units. The study results are based on a sample and not the entire population; thus, we have sampling error. The various origins of sampling error include natural variation among sampling units and variability in measurement of the response. Statistical procedures do require an estimate of the *sampling error.*

Odd is the ratio of the probability of an event to the probability of a nonevent, for example, flipping a coin and getting a head as an event versus getting tail as the nonevent. For example, the odds of flipping a head is 1:1, as both heads and tail have an equal probability (0.50/0.50) of occurrence. If you now consider a six-sided die and asked about the odds of rolling a specific value, say three, the odds now become 1:5 (probability of a three is one possible outcome out of six total outcomes [0.1667] versus five of six [0.8333] other values, for the ratio of 0.1667/0.8333 = 0.20 or 1:5). In other words, the nonevent is five times more likely than the event.

Odds ratio is the ratio of the odds of an event for a particular group versus the odds of that event for a different group.

Logit is the natural logarithm of the odds. It is the natural log (probability of event/probability of nonevent).

$$logit(p) = \ln\left(\frac{p}{1-p}\right)$$

Bernoulli trial is a single random event for which there are two and only two possible outcomes. These outcomes are mutually exclusive. The custom is to define one outcome termed a success and assigned the score of 1, while the other is a failure and given the score of 0. For example, a patient survived the operation versus not is a Bernoulli trial.

Binomial random variable is a sum of independent Bernoulli trials.

Binomial distribution is used for handling the errors associated with regression models for binary/dichotomous responses (i.e., yes/no, dead/alive) in the same way that the normal distribution is used in simple or multiple linear regression models.

Binary models often use logistic regression models, because of their many desirable properties such as interpretation in terms of the odds (Hosmer & Lemeshow, 1989; McCullagh & Nelder, 1989; Cox & Snell, 1989; Pregibon, 1981). Other less commonly used binomial models include normit/probit and complimentary log-log.

Maximum likelihood is a method of finding the smallest possible difference between the observed and the predicted (model) values. We assume the probability of the outcome has a known distribution. Once this smallest value has been obtained, then the best solution for the parameter is the "negative two log likelihood" (Cohen et al. (2003); Hosmer & Lemeshow, 1989).

Exponential family—a set of distributions which has great flexibility in the relations between the variance as related to the mean of the response variable. They provide natural links between the mean of the response variable and the covariates in the model (McCullagh & Nelder, 1989). Some examples are binomial, Poisson, and normal distribution.

Canonical link—once the distribution in the exponential family is written in a certain form, it provides a link (called the canonical link) that relates the mean of the response distribution to the covariates.

Hessian matrix was developed in the nineteenth century by the German mathematician Ludwig Otto Hesse and later named after him. It is a square symmetric matrix with cells consisting of the second derivatives of the function of interest.

Likelihood function is a function of the parameters of a statistical model, defined as follows: The *likelihood* of a set of parameter values, given some observed outcomes, is equal to the *probability* of those observed outcomes, given those parameter values. The nonstatistical world usually sees "likelihood" as a synonym for "probability." However, asking "If I were to flip a fair coin 100 times, what is the *probability* of it landing heads-up every time?" and asking "Given that I have flipped a coin 100 times and it has landed heads-up 100 times, what is the *likelihood* that the coin is fair?" are two very different questions that show how improper it is to use "likelihood" and "probability" interchangeably. The likelihood function indicates how likely a parameter value is in light of the observed data.

A *prospective study* or cohort study may involve the selection of two comparable groups, one for treatment and the other for control, to be observed over a period of time. The result of it is the outcome for each individual according to whether or not the event being studied is recorded. A *prospective* study is often conducted in order to determine if there is an association between certain covariates and the occurrence (probability) of a particular event. This relationship can then be investigated through the fit of certain generalized linear models with probit, logit, or complimentary log-log links.

Retrospective or *case control* studies are good for studying rare conditions because they are relatively inexpensive, the sample sizes do not have to be extremely large, they require less time than prospective studies because the outcome being studied has already occurred, and they can simultaneously look at multiple risk factors. A *retrospective* study is an etiologic (etiologic treatment of a disease seeks to remove or correct its cause) study in which comparisons are made between individuals who have a particular event, known as cases, and individuals who do not have the event, known as controls. A sample of cases is selected from a population of individuals who have the event being studied, and a sample of controls is selected from individuals who do not have the event. Information about the factors, which might be associated with the event, is obtained retrospectively for each person in the study (Wang & Carroll, 1999).

3.3 Exploratory Analyses

While using a simple linear regression to test the administrators' rehospitalization hypothesis might seem like a good idea at first, there are significant challenges when analyzing the collected data in that way. Many studies have mistakenly used simple linear regression for such tasks when a logistic regression would be better suited. Therefore, let us consider the Medicare data and explore using simple linear (Fig. 3.1). Figure 3.1 provides a plot of predicted values from a linear regression of rehospitalization using the number of diagnoses.

Figure 3.2 provides a plot of predicted probabilities from a simple linear regression of rehospitalization using the number of diagnoses, length of stay, and the presence of atherosclerosis.

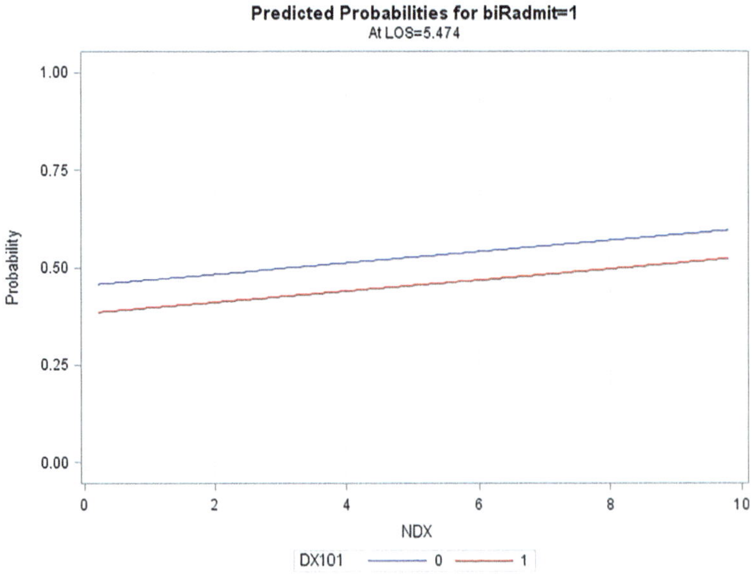

Fig. 3.1 Predicted probabilities for readmission versus NDX (number of diseases)

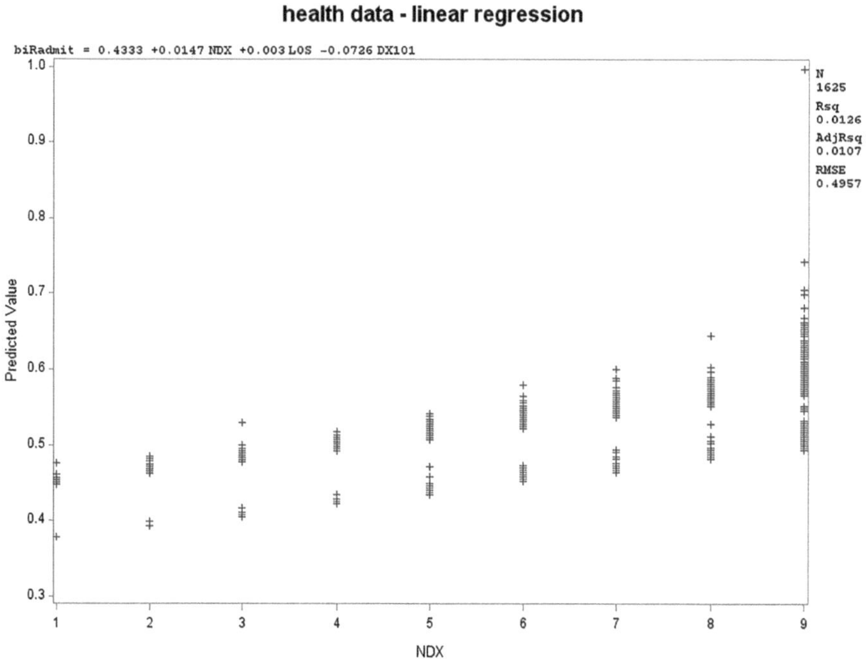

Fig. 3.2 Predicted probabilities on a linear scale versus NDX (number of disease)

Source	DF	Sum of Squares	Mean Square	F Value	Pr > F
Model	3	5.06901	1.68967	6.88	0.0001
Error	1621	398.37714	0.24576		
Corrected Tot	1624	403.44615			
Root MSE	0.49574	R-Square	0.0126		
Dependent Mean	0.54154	Adj R-Sq	0.0107		
Coeff Var	91.54326				

Parameter Estimates

Variable	DF	Parameter Estimate	Standard Error	t Value	Pr > |t|
Intercept	1	0.43330	0.04632	9.36	<.0001
DX101	1	-0.07259	0.03127	-2.32	0.0204
NDX	1	0.01468	0.00620	2.37	0.0181
LOS	1	0.00304	0.00208	1.46	0.1433

Comments Of course, whatever you put into the computer will produce results, but the interpretation is what makes the difference. We have a linear model based on ordinary least squares as $\hat{P}_{biRadmit=1} = 0.433 - 0.073\text{DX101} + 0.015\text{NDX} + 0.003\text{LOS}$.

The challenges with using a simple linear regression on binary data are as follows:

1. There are no limits on the values predicted by a linear regression, so the predicted response (mean) might be less than 0 or greater than 1, which is clearly outside the realm of possible values for a response probability.
2. The variance of the outcomes for each subpopulation is different and is not constant. The variance is a function of the mean. As the mean changes from subpopulation to subpopulation, the variance will also change. Hence, we cannot claim homogeneity of variance (as required) in this situation as we can in ordinary linear regression.
3. While using a weighted linear regression model might seem to solve the issue, we would still be faced with the problem of predicted values not lying between zero and one.

The problems encountered while trying to fit a simple linear regression model can be best addressed by fitting a logistic regression model. Logistic regression models describe the relationship between a binary or categorical response variable and a set of predictor variables. In this chapter, we concentrate on independent binary responses, while the rest of the book examines correlated binary observations.

Consider the following system where **X** denotes a set of input variables in the system and Y denotes the output variable (Fig. 3.3). Here, **X** represents multiple input variables, also referred to as independent, explanatory, concomitant, and predictor variables, or drivers or factors depending on the discipline or topic. Our known information, denoted by **X**, can consist of a quantitative or continuous variable, a binary variable, or a categorical variable. The input of the system may consist of all or some combination of these different types of variables. The binary output variable denoted by Y is referred to as the response or dependent variable. Fig. 3.3 illustrates that given a set of p explanatory variables where $\mathbf{X} = (X_1, X_2, \ldots X_p)$, the average value of Y can be explained by some or all of these variables. In this chapter, we fit a standard logistic regression model:

$$\log\left(\frac{P_1}{P_0}\right) = \beta_0 X_0 + \beta_1 X_1 + \ldots \beta_I X_I$$

where P_1 and P_0 denote the probability of a favorable response and an unfavorable response, respectively, and β_i denote the ith regression coefficients (providing the weights) associated with the X_i for $i = 1, \ldots I$ and where X_0 is defined as the constant value of one.

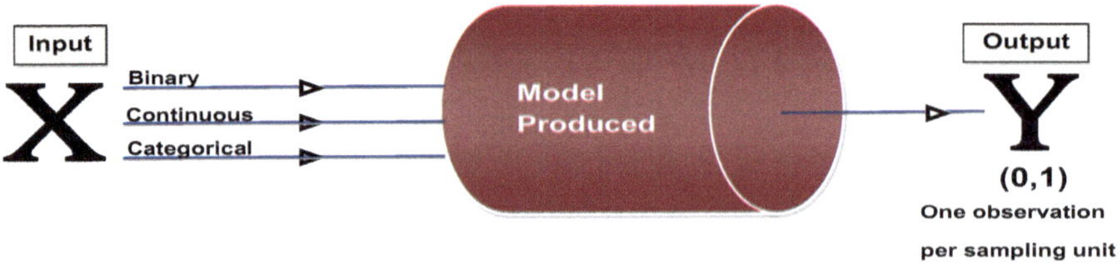

Fig. 3.3 Modeling a binary response

3.4 Statistical Models

The logistic regression model is a type of predictive modeling that can be used when the response variable is binary, meaning that there are only two possible outcomes such as live/die, disease/no disease, purchase/no purchase, win/lose, etc. In short, logistic regression models are used when we want to model the probability of a certain outcome. In fact, we are modeling the mean of the response (which is the probability in the case of binary variables). A logistic regression model can be applied to response variables with more than two categories; however, those cases, though referred to from time to time in this book, are not the focus but can surely be explored further for independent observations (Agresti, 2002).

As the responses are not on a continuous measure and as such are not continuous, the use of logistic regression differs somewhat from the well-known linear regression, because, while in both cases we are modeling the mean, the mean in regression lies anywhere between $(-\infty, +\infty)$ whereas the mean (or the probability) in logistic regression lies between [0, 1]. Thus, we are predicting the probability that *Y* is equal to 1 (rather than 0) given certain cases of the predictors $X_1, \ldots, X_p$. It is important to make the distinction between these logistic and linear regression models so we can think about how the observed data may be 0 or 1, but the predicted value may lie between [0, 1]. For example, we might try to predict the probability of whether a patient will live or die based on the patient's age as well as the number of years of experience his or her operating physician has.

The general form of the logistic regression model is

$$\log\left(\frac{p_I}{1-p_I}\right) = \beta_0 + \beta_1 X_1 + \ldots \beta_I X_I$$

where p_I is the probability that Y = 1 (the event), given $X_1 \ldots X_I$ are the covariates (predictors) and β_I i = 1, 2…p are known as the regression coefficients, which have to be estimated from the data. Logistic regression model forms a linear combination of the explanatory variables to impact the logit, which is log {probability of event/probability nonevent}. On the logit scale, the relation is linear. On the probability scale, it has the shape of an S, and on the odds scale, it is also nonlinear.

3.4.1 Probability

Let probability p_I denote success and $1 - p_I$ denote failure with the results constrained to lie between 0 and 1. On the probability scale, we define

$$p_I = \frac{\exp[\beta_0 + \beta_1 X_1 + \ldots \beta_I X_I]}{1 + \exp[\beta_0 + \beta_1 X_1 + \ldots + \beta_I X_I]}$$

The constraints of $0 \leq p_I \leq 1$ make it impossible to construct a linear equation for predicting probabilities.

3.4.2 Odds

On the odds scale, define

$$\frac{p_1}{1-p_1} = \exp\left[\beta_0 + \beta_1 X_1 + \ldots + \beta_I X_I\right]$$

They are constrained by $0 \leq \frac{p_1}{1-p_1} < \infty$, with 1 as the point for which both outcomes are equally likely. Odds are asymmetric. If we invert the odds or consider the two outcomes as switched, each value in the range 0 to 1 is transformed by taking its inverse (1/value) to a value in the range 1 to +∞. For example, if the odds of rehospitalization are 1/4, the odds of not being rehospitalized are 4/1.

3.4.3 Logits

On the logit scale, define

$$\log\left(\frac{p_1}{1-p_1}\right) = \beta_0 + \beta_1 X_1 + \ldots + \beta_p X_p.$$

On this scale, we have linearity. The logits are symmetric. They lie in the range −∞ to +∞. The value that is equally likely for both outcomes is 0. If the identification of the two outcomes is switched, the log odds are multiplied by −1, since log (a/b) = −log (b/a). For example, if the log odds of rehospitalization are 0.6026, the log odds of not being rehospitalized are −0.6026. As the probability of an outcome increases, the odds and log odds also increase. The log odds of an event relays equally the same message as the probability of the event, so if a certain predictor has a positive impact on the logit, then it has the same directional effect on the odds. When the log odds take on any value between −∞ and +∞, the coefficients form a logistic regression equation that can be interpreted in the usual way, meaning that they represent the change in log odds of the response per unit change in the predictor.

3.4.4 Logistic Regression Versus Ordinary Least Squares

In this section, we addressed the differences between using a linear regression model (i.e., obtaining estimates through ordinary least squares) on binary data as opposed to logistic regression model and presented a summary of their comparatives. When fitting logistic regression models, the researcher is predicting the probability of a binary outcome (the mean). In a logistic regression model, the errors follow a logistic distribution, whereas in the ordinary least squares model, the errors are normally distributed. The logistic regression model takes the logit of the probability of a favorable outcome and provides an explanation for its variation through a set of possible input variables. In such case, the underlying distribution is Bernoulli; the link between the probability (mean of the distribution) and the covariates is logit. Thus, the logistic regression belongs to a class of models called generalized linear models.

Unlike ordinary linear regression models, logistic regression models do not assume that the relationship between the covariates and the mean of the response variable is a linear one. Nor does it assume that the response variable or the error terms are distributed normally. When fitting a logistic regression model, there is no R^2 to gauge the variance accounted for in the overall model (at least not one that has been agreed upon by statisticians). Instead, we rely on a goodness-of-fit chi-square test to indicate how well the logistic regression model fits the data (Agresti, 2002) and Hosmer and Lemeshow's goodness-of-fit (Hosmer & Lemeshow, 1989).

For logistic regression models, the response variable is an indicator of some characteristic, that is, a binary variable, whereas in the ordinary linear least squares regression, the response variable is continuous and hence it cannot have a binomial distribution. Logistic regression is used to determine whether certain factors influence the presence of some characteristics, for example, whether certain characteristics are predictive of the probability that a customer would default on a loan, or the probability of a driver getting in an accident, or the probability of a patient surviving an operation, or probability of a student succeeding in graduate school.

Although the response variable in a logistic regression model is binary, the logistic regression equation, which is a linear equation, does not predict the outcome of the binary variable but rather the probability of the outcome. The importance of the regression coefficients denotes how the specific covariate has predictive capability in the system of variables. Instead of classifying an observation into one group or the other, logistic regression predicts the probability that the binary response is an event. To be precise, the logistic regression equation does not directly predict the probability that the outcome is an event. It predicts the log odds that an observation will have an event outcome with certain characteristics.

3.4.5 *Generalized Linear Models (GLMs)*

A logistic regression model belongs to a class of models referred to as generalized linear models (GLMs). GLMs are defined by three components:

1. A random component that specifies the probability distribution of the response variable. The data are assumed to be as a result of independent observations from a distribution belonging to the exponential family (component 1).
2. A systematic component, which specifies a linear function of the covariate so $\beta_0 + \beta_1 X_1 + \ldots + \beta_p X_p$ (component 2).
3. The link function, which relates a linear combination of predictors (component 2) and the mean of the response variable (component 1).

So, in the use of logistic regression models, component 1 is the binomial distribution with mean *np* and variance $np(1-p)$. Component 2 will be the right side of our model, $\beta_0 + \beta_1 X_1 + \ldots + \beta_p X_p$, and component 3 is the logit that combines *np* and $\beta_0 + \beta_1 X_1 + \ldots + \beta_p X_p$ to result in

$$\log\left(\frac{np_1}{n - np_1}\right) = \beta_0 + \beta_1 X_1 + \ldots + \beta_p X_p.$$

The GLMs provide a unified approach to modeling the mean of a random variable (in this case the probability of the binary variable outcome) with known distribution (Nelder & Wedderburn, 1972). Essentially, a GLM describes how a function of the mean relates linearly to the set of predictors. In particular, we look at the logit link, such that

$$\log\left(\frac{P_1}{P_0}\right) = \beta_0 + \beta_1 X_1 + \ldots + \beta_I X_I$$

where P_1 denotes the probability of the event and P_0 denotes the probability of the nonevent; it links the probability p_1 with the set of $X_i : i = 1, \ldots, I$. The effect of a unit change in x_i changes the log odds by an amount $\hat{\beta}_i$, an estimate of β_i, which is the ith element in the set of parameters. Equivalently, the effect of a unit change in x_i leads to an increase in the odds of a positive response multiplicatively by the factor $\exp(\hat{\beta}_i)$, while other predictors are accounted for. The idea of generalized linear models (McCullagh & Nelder, 1989) provides an extension of linear models, since it allows us to use other distributions which negates the need for the assumptions of normality, constant error variance, and a linear relationship between the covariate effects and the mean.

3.4.6 *Response Probability Distributions*

In GLMs, the response is assumed to possess a probability distribution from the exponential family. That is, the probability density of the response y for continuous response variables, or the probability function for discrete responses, can be expressed in a special form (Dobson & Barnett, 2008). In this form, we can easily determine the mean and variance and the so-called canonical link, a special link obtained when the distribution is written in a certain form, the so-called canonical form.

3.4.7 *Log-Likelihood Functions*

Let the ith observation have a response y_i either one or zero with mean μ_i and dispersion parameter φ. Then for each observation, there is a likelihood function l_i so the joint log-likelihood function is

$$L(\mathrm{y},\mu,\varphi) = \mathrm{Sum}_i \text{ of } \{l_i\},$$

where Sum_i represents the sum of the likelihood function over the independent observations.

3.4.8 Maximum Likelihood Fitting

The aim is to maximize the log-likelihood function $L(\mathrm{y}, \mu, \varphi)$ with respect to the regression parameters. It is useful to note, at this point, that while maximum likelihood estimators have desirable properties, they are not useful for analyzing correlated observations. In most of the remaining pages in this book, we concentrate on correlated data. Therefore, the joint likelihood will be unknown and other methods must be explored. The correlated observations deny us the opportunity to sum the likelihood function.

3.4.9 Goodness-of-Fit

Two statistics that are helpful in assessing the goodness-of-fit of a GLM are the scaled deviance and Pearson's chi-square statistic. For a fixed value of the dispersion parameter φ, the scaled deviance is defined to be twice the difference between the maximum achievable log likelihood and the log likelihood at the maximum likelihood estimates of the regression parameters. The scaled version of both of these statistics, under certain regularity conditions, has a limiting chi-square distribution, with degrees of freedom equal to the number of observations minus the number of parameters estimated. The scaled version can be used as an approximate guide to the goodness-of-fit of a given model. *Use caution before applying these statistics to ensure that all the conditions for the asymptotic distributions hold.* McCullagh and Nelder (1989) advised that differences in deviances for nested models can be better approximated by chi-square distributions than the deviances can themselves. In cases where the dispersion parameter is not known, an estimate can be used to obtain an approximation to the scaled deviance and Pearson's chi-square statistic. One strategy is to fit a model that contains a sufficient number of parameters so that all systematic variation is removed, estimate φ from this model, and then use this estimate in computing the scaled deviance of sub models. The deviance or Pearson's chi-square divided by its degrees of freedom is sometimes used as an estimate of the dispersion parameter φ. For example, since the limiting chi-square distribution of the scaled deviance has $\mathrm{n} - \mathrm{p}$ degrees of freedom, where n is the number of observations and p is the number of parameters, equating scaled deviance to its mean and solving for φ yield $\widehat{\varphi} = \frac{\text{deviance}}{\mathrm{n}-\mathrm{p}} = \phi = D/(n-p)$. Similarly, an estimate of φ based on Pearson's chi-square is $\widehat{\varphi} = \mathrm{X}^2/(\mathrm{n}-\mathrm{p})$.

3.4.10 Other Fit Statistics

The Akaike information criterion (AIC) is a measure of goodness of model fit that balances model fit against model simplicity, no variables included. An alternative form is the corrected

$$\mathrm{AICC} = \mathrm{AIC} + \frac{2p(p-1)}{n-p-1}$$

where n denotes the total number of observations used and p is the number of parameters. The Bayesian information criterion (BIC) is a similar measure of goodness-of-fit (Akaike, 1981). Simonoff (2003) provides information for using AIC, AICC, and BIC with generalized linear models. These criteria are useful in selecting among regression models, with smaller values representing better model fit.

3.4.11 Assumptions for Logistic Regression Model

When fitting a standard binary logistic regression model, there are important assumptions that need to be satisfied: Observations are assumed independent, and the effect of any clustering is ignored. If there is a violation of the independence assumption, then this may result in incorrect inferences about the regression coefficient or inefficient estimates of regression coefficients.

3.4.12 Interpretation of Coefficients

The $\hat{\beta}_i$ represents the change in $\log\left(\frac{\hat{p}}{1-\hat{p}}\right)$ with one unit change in X_i while the other X variables are held constant or, equivalently, the change in the odds ratio with one unit change in $e^{\hat{\beta}_i}$.

3.4.13 Interpretation of Odds Ratio (OR)

In exploring the interpretation of the odds ratio, let us consider two cases, one where X_i is binary and one when it is continuous:

When X_i is binary, consider.

	$X_i = 1$	$X_i = 0$
Y = 1	$P_{(Y=1\ for\ X_i=1)}$	$P_{(Y=1\ for\ X_i=0)}$
Y = 0	$P_{(Y=0\ for\ X_i=1)}$	$P_{(Y=0\ for\ X_i=0)}$

$$OR = \frac{P_{(Y=1\ for\ X_i=1)}P_{(Y=0\ for\ X_i=0)}}{P_{(Y=0\ for\ X_i=1)}P_{(Y=1\ for\ X_i=0)}}$$

If we were to take the logarithm of OR, we would see that it is the difference of two logistic functions, and hence, an estimate of OR is the partial regression coefficient $e^{\hat{\beta}_i}$ when all other predictors are held constant. Thus, the log of the odds ratio is the β_i.

When X_i is continuous, then consider a particular value and that value plus one.

	X_i = 1 + certain value	X_i = a certain value
Y = 1	$P_{(Y=1\ for\ X_i=1+\text{a certain value})}$	$P_{(Y=1\ for\ X_i=\text{a certain value})}$
Y = 0	$P_{(Y=0\ for\ X_i=1+\text{a certain value})}$	$P_{(Y=0\ for\ X_i=\text{a certain value})}$

Thus, an estimate of *OR* is the partial regression coefficient $e^{\hat{\beta}_i}$ when all other predictors are held constant. Thus, the log of the odds ratio is the β_i.

3.4.14 Model Fit

We use chi-square as a measure of model fit. It is the comparison of the observed values to the expected (model) values. The bigger the difference (or "deviance") of the observed values from the expected values, the poorer the fit of the model. Therefore, we want a "small chi-square" if possible. Small in this case is measured by the size of the p-value. As we add more variables to the equation, the deviance should get smaller, indicating an improvement in fit. However, more variables bring additional challenges.

Instead of using the deviance to judge the overall fit of a model, we can compare the fit of the model with and without the predictor(s). This is similar to the change in R^2 (when fitting normal regression models) when another variable has been added to the equation. But here, we expect the deviance to decrease because the degree of error in prediction decreases as we add another variable. To conduct such comparisons, we compare the deviance with just the intercept to the deviance when the new predictor or predictors have been added. The difference between these two deviance values is often referred to as G^2 (Hosmer & Lemeshow, 1989).

While there are several measures to answer how well the model fits, there is still debate on what makes a good measure. Measures are either predictive in nature and goodness-of-fit tests (such as the Pearson chi-square). The Hosmer and Lemeshow test is shown to have some serious problems, since its result can depend on the number of groups. The measures based on Tjur (2009) and McFadden R-square (McFadden, 1974) are some preferred by many for certain reasons. The Tjur statistic has upper bound of 1.0 and bears some resemblance to coefficient of determination for normal linear data.

3.4.15 Null Hypothesis

The statistical null hypothesis is that the simultaneous effects of the predictors do not impact the probability of the response. This means that on the logit scale, the regression coefficient for the linear fit has a value of zero. There are several different ways of obtaining and estimating the p-value associated with the hypothesis. The Wald chi-square is fairly popular, but it may yield inaccurate results with small sample sizes. The likelihood ratio method may be better alternative because it uses the difference between the probability of obtaining the observed results under the logistic regression model and as opposed to the probability of obtaining the observed results in a model with no relationship between the response and covariates (Allison, 2012).

3.4.16 Predicted Probabilities

When modeling a binary response and obtaining predicted probabilities based on a fitted binary model, it is common to overlook the fact that predicted probabilities might differ with respect to the nature of the data (prospective or retrospective) used to fit the model. The difference in the predicted probabilities will depend on the inclusion probability, the probability of being in the sample based on its presence in the population (Fang et al., 2015). They fitted probit, logit, and complimentary log-log to retrospective data knowing that only the logit was appropriate for such data, if we are interested in predicting probabilities. They found that, in all three models, with an inclusion probability of 14%, the predicted probability based on retrospective data was different from what it should have been if perceived as prospective data. It is crucial to understand the difference between predicted probabilities presented based on a retrospective study and predicted probabilities presented based on a prospective study, especially in the context of binary models. In particular, if the number of events to nonevents ratio in the sample is not the same as that in the population, then fitting models based on retrospective data will present certain challenges regarding predicted probabilities. In particular, if the inclusion probability for an event is larger than the inclusion probability for a nonevent, then the estimated predicted probabilities in retrospective studies are larger than in prospective studies. The magnitude of the predictive probabilities for the logit, complimentary log-log link, and the probit link model in the analysis of prospective data as opposed to retrospective data is crucial. In addition, the predictive probabilities based on retrospective and prospective probabilities differ based on the inclusion probabilities. Thus, for the binary links based on logit, probit, and complimentary log-log, the magnitudes of the predicted probabilities based on retrospective versus prospective are not the same. Moreover, with these links, if the inclusion probability for an event is equal to the inclusion probability for a nonevent, then the predictive probabilities are the same regardless of whether the data are sampled prospectively or retrospectively. If the inclusion probability for an event is larger than the inclusion probability for a nonevent, then the estimated probabilities in retrospective studies are larger than those from prospective studies. In particular, if the ratios of the events to the nonevents in the sample are not in the same ratio as in the population, then fitting models based on retrospective data cannot use the predicted probabilities unless they are adjusted.

A predicted probability can be found for any combination of covariate values. In addition, confidence intervals for the predicted probabilities can be determined, but they are expected to be wide as they will incorporate variability for all of the beta coefficients in the model. Some researchers have suggested providing the p-values for the beta coefficients to indicate whether the covariates contribute statistically (statistical significance) and predicted probabilities (without CI) to show what that contribution means (practical significance).

Just as we might be concerned about predicting beyond the scope of the data in linear regression model, there is a danger in using covariate values that are far from the observed values in logistic regression. Some researchers suggested that our focus should remain on model subjects or others of particular interest and then vary just a few covariate values to demonstrate the implications of the model (Oken et al., 2009).

3.4.17 Computational Issues Encountered with Logistic Regression

1. Failure to Converge

If the different covariates have certain values, you may have problems with obtaining regression coefficient estimates and may get a message of "failure to converge." The covariate values are important to the makeup of the so-called Hessian matrix that is used to guide the convergence process. If the Hessian matrix is singular (unable to invert), the logistic regression procedure will be unsuccessful, and a warning message will be displayed.

2. Complete and Quasi-Complete Separation of Values

The estimation of the regression coefficients may also encounter complete separation, a condition where one predictor or a linear combination of predictors perfectly predicts the target value. For example, consider a situation where every value of the response variable is 0 if a certain predictor is less than 10, and every value is 1 if the predictor is greater than 10. The value of response, then, can be perfectly predicted by checking if the predictor is less than or greater than 10. In this case, it is impossible to compute the maximum likelihood values for the regression parameters because the slope of the logistic function would be infinite. At the beginning of each logistic regression analysis, a check should be made for complete separation on each predictor variable. If complete separation is detected, a report (computer output) will be generated with some procedures but not with others (Allison, 2008). The estimation of the regression coefficient may also encounter quasi-complete separation, a condition when values of the target variable overlap or are tied at a single value, or only a few values, of a predictor variable. The analysis may not always check for quasi-complete separation, but the symptoms are extremely large calculated values for the regression parameters or large standard errors. The analysis also may fail to converge. If complete or quasi-complete separation is detected, the predictor variable(s) showing separation should be removed from the analysis (Webb et al., 2004).

3.5 Analysis of Data

In this chapter, we will look at situations involving Bernoulli trials where the sampling units are independent, each unit provides one observation, and the outcome is binary. We will examine a *Medicare* dataset based on rehospitalization and use SAS, SPSS, R, and STATA to analyze the data.

3.5.1 *Medicare Data*

We considered the Medicare data (Sect. 1.7) and modeled the probability of rehospitalization after the first visit using the number of procedures, length of stay, and the presence of coronary atherosclerosis as factors that would influence rehospitalization within 30 days of a patient's release from the hospital. There are 1625 patients in the dataset with complete information. We use the *Medicare* dataset to demonstrate how to fit a logistic regression model, test hypotheses, and interpret the data. Our response is binary, meaning that a patient is either rehospitalized or not rehospitalized within 30 days after discharge. We refer to this as *biRadmit* denoting readmittance. The predictors are the number of prescriptions [NDX], length of stay [LOS], and whether or not the patient has coronary atherosclerosis [DX101]. We used SAS, SPSS, R, and STATA to conduct the fit of the standard logistic regression model. For the fit to the binary data, we had three choices. We could fit the data with the model using the logit scale, or the odds scale, or the probability scale. Thus, we had

$$logit(P_i) = \beta_0 + \beta_1 NDX_i + \beta_2 LOS_i + \beta_3 DX101_i$$

$$\frac{P_i}{[1-P_i]} = e^{\beta_0 + \beta_1 NDX_i + \beta_2 LOS_i + \beta_3 DX101_i}$$

$$P_i = \frac{e^{\beta_0 + \beta_1 NDX_i + \beta_2 LOS_i + \beta_3 DX101_i}}{1 - e^{\beta_0 + \beta_1 NDX_i + \beta_2 LOS_i + \beta_3 DX101_i}}$$

The advantage of using the logit scale for interpretation is that the relationship between the logit and the predictors is a linear one. However, it is just as convenient to state things in terms of probabilities. We must keep in mind that the relationship between the probabilities and the predictors is not a linear relationship. In fact, logistic regression models on the probability scale are at times considered nonlinear models.

3.5.2 *Analysis of Medicare Data with SAS Computing*

SAS Program

```
Data mydata; set perm.Anhdata; run;
where time=1;
ID = _N_;
run;
proc means data = mydata mean std min max N;
var biRadmit NDX LOS DX101;
run;
```

Comments Proc means is a SAS procedure that provides the summary of the data at for time = 1.

SAS Output

The MEANS procedure

Variable	Label	Mean	Std.dev	Minimum	Maximum	N
biRadmit	biRadmit	0.5415385	0.4984250	0	1.0000	1625
NDX	NDX	7.2523077	2.118786	1.000	9.0000	1625
LOS	LOS	5.4738462	6.2967042	0	142.0000	1625
DX101	DX101	0.2049231	0.4037697	0	1.0000	1625

Comment The mean of the binary responses (biRadmit) is 0.542 (when rounding) which is the percentage of patients responding with a "1" that they had been rehospitalized within 30 days.

SAS Program

```
/* Other Features of Proc Logistic */
* CLASS statement, for illustration purpose ;
proc logistic data = mydata ;
 class DX101 (ref='0') /param = ref;
 model biRadmit (event='1') = DX101 NDX LOS ;
run;
* CONTRAST statement, for illustration purpose;
proc logistic data = mydata ;
  class DX101 /param = glm ;
  model biRadmit (event='1') = DX101 NDX LOS;
  contrast '0 vs 1 of DX101' DX101 1 -1 / estimate;
run;
```

Comment The event = ‘1’ allows us to model “1” so that probability of the event = 1 is in the numerator. So, we have $\log(P_{biRadmit=1}/P_{biRadmit=0})$ instead of $\log(P_{biRadmit=0}/P_{biRadmit=1})$. The CLASS statements identify which level will be the reference level.

SAS Output

```
                    Model Information
Dataset                               WORK.MYDATA
Response Variable                       biRadmit
Number of Response Levels                  2
Model                                   binary logit
Optimization Technique                  Fisher's scoring
```

Comment We are fitting a binary logit. We use the Fisher’s scoring method to obtain the estimates of the regression coefficient.

```
Number of Observations Read        1625
Number of Observations Used        1625
```

Comment There are no missing values. We were able to use all 1625 observations.

Response Profile

Ordered Value	biRadmit	Total Frequency
1	0	745
2	1	880

Comment There are 880 cases with output 1 and 745 cases with output 0. Probability modeled is biRadmit = '1'. We are modeling the probability of the outcome which is 1, thus $\log(P_{biRadmit=1}/P_{biRadmit=0})$.

Model Convergence Status

Convergence criterion (GCONV=1E-8) satisfied.

Model Fit Statistics

Criterion	Intercept Only	Intercept and Covariates
AIC	2243.500	2228.875
SC	2248.893	2250.448
-2 Log L	2241.500	2220.875

Comment There are three statistics that tell us about the fit—the difference between "Intercept Only" and "Intercept" and the "covariates." We have AIC = (Akaike information criterion) and SC (=Schwarz criterion) and −2log L = (− twice log likelihood), where smaller values represent a model that is a better fit to the data. The differences in the model fit statistics are as follows:

	Difference
AIC	14.625
SC	1.555
−2 log L	20.625

Comment The difference serves as a joint test for the significance of the three covariates.

Testing Global Null Hypothesis: BETA = 0

Test	Chi-square	DF	Pr > ChiSq
Likelihood Ratio	20.6254	3	0.0001
Score	20.4170	3	0.0001
Wald	20.0557	3	0.0002

Comment The three tests (likelihood ratio, score, Wald) are significant. We see that from the very small p-values, DX101, NDX, and LOS together have a jointly significant effect on rehospitalization.

The Logistic Procedure

Type 3 Analysis of Effects

Effect	DF	Wald Chi-square	Pr > ChiSq
DX101	1	5.2328	0.0222
NDX	1	5.1968	0.0226
LOS	1	2.1013	0.1472

Comment The added effect of each of the three covariates shows that DX101 ($p = 0.0222$) and NDX ($p = 0.0222$) are significant but LOS is not. [We used $\alpha = 0.05$ as a yardstick for comparison for significance.]

Analysis of Maximum Likelihood Estimates

Parameter	DF	Estimate	Standard Error	Wald Chi-square	Pr > ChiSq
Intercept	1	-0.2699	0.1876	2.0693	0.1503
DX101	1	-0.2903	0.1269	5.2328	0.0222
NDX	1	0.0580	0.0254	5.1968	0.0226
LOS	1	0.0141	0.00974	2.1013	0.1472

Comment The logistic regression model is best represented by

$$\log\left(\hat{P}_{biRadmit=1} / \hat{P}_{biRadmit=0}\right) = -0.270 - 0.290\text{DX101} + 0.058\text{NDX} + 0.014\text{LOS}$$

These beta coefficients are estimated through the method of maximum likelihood. To obtain such estimates, we have to assume a distribution. We assumed the Bernoulli trial, which led to the binomial distribution (the sum of independent Bernoulli trials). The intercept has a parameter estimate of −0.270. This is the estimated logit when DX101 = 0, LOS = 0, and NDX = 0, meaning that the patient had no diagnosis, was not hospitalized, and had no coronary atherosclerosis. This really makes no sense here. There are times when the intercept is not interpretable, and this is one such time. The coefficient for the binary variable DX101 is −0.290, which means that for patients with coronary atherosclerosis versus those without coronary atherosclerosis, the expected change in the log of odds is 0.290 given that NDX and LOS stay fixed. In other words, if two patients are compared and the only thing that differs is that one has DX101 (coronary atherosclerosis) and the other does not, then the difference is 0.290 on the logit scale.

Odds Ratio Estimates

Effect	Point Estimate	95% Wald Confidence Limits	
DX101 1 vs 0	0.748	0.583	0.959
NDX	1.060	1.008	1.114
LOS	1.014	0.995	1.034

Comment We can also interpret the results on the scale of the odds ratio. The odds for a DX101 patient are exp(−0.2699 − 0.2903 + 0.0580 + 0.0141) = 0.6138, and the odds for a non-DX101 patient are exp(−0.2699 + 0.0580 + 0.0141) = 0.8205. Therefore, taking the ratio of these two odds, we get the odds ratio for DX101 = 1 versus DX101 = 0 as 0.6138/0.8205 = 0.7481. We are also given the 95% Wald confidence limits as [0.583, 0.959]. In terms of probabilities, the probability for a DX101 patient to be rehospitalized (all other things being equal) is (0.6138)/(1 + 0.6138) =0.3803. The probability for non-DX101 is 1-0.3803 = 0.6197. One should not confuse the adjusted odds ratio, 0.748, which is the conditional, with the unadjusted odds ratio 0.681, {=(567 × 155)/(178 × 725)} = 0.68 computed from the table of frequencies.

Cross Classification of Rehospitalization by DX101

biRadmit	DX101 = 0	DX101 = 1
0	567	178
1	725	155

```
                                            Cumulative  Cumulative
 biRadmit    DX101    Frequency    Percent   Frequency    Percent
-------------------------------------------------------------------
     0          0         567       34.89        567        34.89
     0          1         178       10.95        745        45.85
     1          0         725       44.62       1470        90.46
     1          1         155        9.54       1625       100.00
```

Comment The unadjusted odds ratio is 155*567/725*178 = 0.681, which is different from 0.748 which is computed when all the variables are in the model.

Readmit	DX101 = 0	DX101 = 1
0	567	178
1	725	155

The former is the unadjusted odds ratio while the latter is the adjusted odds ratio. Too often, researchers use the two-variable-at-a-time approach in research to analyze the data, when in fact these covariates all exist simultaneously.

Association of Predicted Probabilities and Observed Responses

```
Percent Concordant       56.8     Somers' D     0.157
Percent Discordant       41.1      Gamma        0.161
Percent Tied              2.1      Tau-a        0.078
Pairs                  655600        c          0.579
```

Comment Once the model is fitted, we can then go back and compute the probability of rehospitalization for each patient. Those so-called predicted probabilities will not be 0 or 1 but will lie between [0, 1]. To make comparisons (though not usually advisable) among the given responses in the data, we need to dichotomize those predicted probabilities. We can do that based on 0.50 or based on the prior probabilities observed in the dataset, 880/1625 = 0.5415 (as obtained from the response profile). However, in this case, SAS used 0.50 and obtained a 2 by 2 table of observed versus predicted probabilities. The percent concordant and discordant as well as the other values are computed from that table.

Contrast estimation and testing results by row

Contrast	Type	Row	Estimate	Standarderror	Alpha	Confidence limits		Wald chi-square	Pr > ChiSq
0 VS 1	PARAM	1	0.2903	0.1269	0.05	0.0416	0.5391	5.2328	0.0222

Comment Using the contrast statement in the second program allows for a specific test of model parameters using an asymptotic Wald chi-square test of the null hypothesis, showing that a linear combination of the coefficients is zero. In this case, we test whether or not the patient has NDX101 = 0 versus NDX101 = 1.

SAS PROGRAM

```
* TEST Statement;
proc logistic data = mydata ;
model biRadmit (event='1') = DX101 NDX LOS;
  test_LOS_NDX: test LOS, NDX;  * tested on the joint effect of
LOS and NDX. ;
  test_equal: test LOS = NDX;    * tested on the hypothesis that
the effect of     LOS and NDX are the same on rehospitalization;
run;
```

SAS Output

The output consists of the previously stated output plus the following:

Linear Hypotheses Testing Results

Label	Wald Chi-square	DF	Pr > ChiSq
test_LOS_NDX	10.5609	2	0.0051
test_equal	2.1314	1	0.1443

Comment We have first the test that $\beta_{los} = \beta_{ndx} = 0$ that is the joint effect of LOS and NDX equal zero. A p-value of 0.0051 shows that the joint effect is significant. The test $\beta_{los} = \beta_{ndx}$ has a p-value with 0.1443, meaning the effects of LOS are not significantly different from the effects of NDX in the model.

SAS Program

```
* LACKFIT and RSQUARE Option;
proc logistic data = mydata;
model biRadmit(event='1') =DX101 LOS NDX / rsq lackfit;
run;
```

Comment This provides a test of the model we refer to as lack of fit and gives a so-called R-square value.

SAS Output

The output consists of the previously stated output plus the following:

R-square	0.0126	Max-rescaled R-square	0.0169

Partition for the Hosmer and Lemeshow Test

Group	Total	biRadmit = 1 Observed	biRadmit = 1 Expected	biRadmit = 0 Observed	biRadmit = 0 Expected
1	162	73	69.66	89	92.34
2	170	78	81.76	92	88.24
3	163	76	82.41	87	80.59
4	162	84	85.23	78	76.77
5	168	92	91.91	76	76.09
6	189	93	106.87	96	82.13
7	157	95	90.30	62	66.70
8	149	89	86.73	60	62.27
9	175	118	103.73	57	71.27
10	130	82	81.42	48	48.58

Hosmer and Lemeshow Goodness-of-Fit Test

Chi-square	DF	Pr > ChiSq
11.3524	8	0.1825

Comment The model is a good fit. The R^2 statistic that is produced in the MODEL line is a generalized coefficient of determination proposed by Cox and Snell (1989). The max-rescaled R^2 is adjusted to have a maximum value of 1.0, as proposed by Nagelkerke (1991). Since the so-called response variable is binary, any attempt to look at the predicted values versus the observed values will not result in useful information regarding the fit of the model. However, through the Hosmer and Lemeshow goodness-of-fit test, we can decide whether the model is a good fit. A p-value of 0.1825 suggests that there is no significant residual after this model was fitted.

PNUM_R	biRadmit	NDX	LOS	DX101	PRE_1
127	0	9	6	1	0.51161
560	1	9	8	0	0.59025
746	1	6	12	0	0.56156
750	0	9	6	0	0.58341
1117	0	9	5	1	0.50808
1395	1	9	6	0	0.58341
1568	1	8	2	0	0.55535
2076	1	9	8	1	0.51866
2390	0	7	2	0	0.54098

2413	0	9	17	0	0.62060
3008	0	5	2	0	0.51208
3123	1	9	3	0	0.57308
3710	1	6	3	0	0.53007
3970	0	9	1	0	0.56615
3982	0	7	1	0	0.53748
4236	0	9	5	0	0.57997
4581	1	9	3	1	0.50102
4873	0	9	1	1	0.49396
5387	0	3	3	0	0.48662
6255	0	9	5	0	0.57997
7497	0	8	4	0	0.56231
7599	0	7	4	1	0.47558

3.5.3 Analysis of Medicare Data with SPSS Computing

SPSS Program Code

```
LOGISTIC REGRESSION VARIABLES biRadmit
  /METHOD=ENTER NDX DX101 LOS
  /PRINT=SUMMARY
  /CRITERIA=PIN(0.05) POUT(0.10) ITERATE(20) CUT(0.5).
```

SPSS Pull-Down Menu

```
Step 1:
Click "Analyze" on the toolbar
Select "Regression"
Click "Binary Logistic"
Step 2:
Select the dependent variable in the left column
Click the arrow next to "Dependent"
Select the independent variables in the left column
Click the arrow next to "Covariates"
Click "OK" at the bottom of the window
```

SPSS Output

Case processing summary

Unweighted cases[a]		N	Percent
Selected cases	Included in analysis	1625	100.0
	Missing cases	0	0.0
	Total	1625	100.0
Unselected cases		0	0.0
Total		1625	100.0

[a]If weight is in effect, see the classification table for the total number of cases

Comment

All observations were used. There were no missing values.

Model summary

Step	−2 Log likelihood	Cox and Snell R-square	Nagelkerke R-square
1	2220.875[a]	0.013	0.017

[a]Estimation terminated at iteration number 3 because parameter estimates changed by less than 0.001

Comment The Cox and Snell and Nagelkerke generalized R^2 values are meant to mimic the R^2 in the regression model for continuous data.

Classification Table[a]

	Observed		Predicted		
			biRadmit		Percentage Correct
			0	1	
Step 1	biRadmit	0	195	550	26.2
		1	163	717	81.5
	Overall percentage				56.1

[a]The cut value is 0.500

Comment The predicted values lie between [0,1]. So any comparisons with the original data require a dichotomization of the predicted probabilities. One such method is to use 0.50 as the cutoff. The classification table depends on the cut point chosen. Some researchers may choose to use 0.54 as the cutoff as it coincides with prior probabilities.

	Variables in the equation						
		B	S.E.	Wald	df	Sig.	Exp(B)
Step 1[a]	NDX	0.058	0.025	5.197	1	0.023	1.060
	DX101	−0.290	0.127	5.233	1	0.022	0.748
	LOS	0.014	0.010	2.101	1	0.147	1.014
	Constant	−0.270	0.188	2.069	1	0.150	0.763

[a]Variable(s) entered on step 1: NDX, DX101, LOS

Comment The B column has the results from the maximum likelihood estimates in the logit scale, and the exp.(B) values give the odds ratio values. Note that SPSS uses three significant digits, so values may appear to be different from other programs but that is due purely to rounding. The logistic regression model is best represented by

$$\log\left(\hat{P}_{biRadmit=1} / \hat{P}_{biRadmit=0}\right) = -0.270 - 0.290\text{DX101} + 0.058\text{NDX} + 0.0141\text{LOS}$$

PNUM_R	biRadmit	NDX	LOS	DX101	PRE_1
127	0	9	6	1	0.51161
560	1	9	8	0	0.59025
746	1	6	12	0	0.56156
750	0	9	6	0	0.58341
1117	0	9	5	1	0.50808
1395	1	9	6	0	0.58341
1568	1	8	2	0	0.55535
2076	1	9	8	1	0.51866
2390	0	7	2	0	0.54098
2413	0	9	17	0	0.62060
3008	0	5	2	0	0.51208
3123	1	9	3	0	0.57308
3710	1	6	3	0	0.53007
3970	0	9	1	0	0.56615
3982	0	7	1	0	0.53748
4236	0	9	5	0	0.57997
4581	1	9	3	1	0.50102
4873	0	9	1	1	0.49396
5387	0	3	3	0	0.48662
6255	0	9	5	0	0.57997
7497	0	8	4	0	0.56231
7599	0	7	4	1	0.47558

These beta coefficients are estimated through the method of maximum likelihood. To obtain such estimates, we had to assume a distribution. We assumed the Bernoulli trial, which led to the binomial distribution (the sum of independent Bernoulli trials). The intercept has a parameter estimate of −0.270. This is the estimated logit when DX101 = 0, LOS = 0, and NDX = 0. It is when the patient had no diagnosis, was not hospitalized, and had no coronary atherosclerosis. This really makes no sense here. There are times when the intercept is not interpretable, and this is one such time. The coefficient for the binary variable DX101 is −0.290. That means that for patients with coronary atherosclerosis versus those without coronary atherosclerosis, the expected change in the log of odds is 0.290 given that NDX and LOS stay fixed. In other words, if two patients were to be compared and the only thing that differs between them is that one has DX101 (coronary atherosclerosis) and the other does not, then the difference is 0.290 on the logit scale. So, a patient with DX101 has a higher chance of being readmitted.

3.5.4 Analysis of Medicare Data with R Computing

R Program

```
> glm.out=glm(biRadmit ~ DX101+LOS+NDX, family=binomial(logit),
data=data2)
> summary(glm.out)
Call: glm(formula = biRadmit ~ DX101 + LOS + NDX, family =
binomial(logit),
    data = data2)
```

R Output

```
Deviance Residuals:
 Min            1Q            Median           3Q           Max
-2.1710        -1.2412        0.9995          1.0794       1.3905
Coefficients:
               Estimate      Std. Error      z value     Pr(>|z|)
(Intercept)   -0.269890      0.187617        -1.439       0.1503
DX101         -0.290320      0.126914        -2.288       0.0222*
LOS            0.014120      0.009741         1.450       0.1472
NDX            0.057994      0.025440         2.280       0.0226*
```

Signif. codes: 0 '***' 0.001 '**' 0.01 '*' 0.05 '.' 0.1 '' 1.

Comment The estimate column contains the maximum likelihood estimates based on the logit scale. Note that the test statistics are z-scores, or the square root of the Wald chi-square statistics in the type 3 analysis of effects table in SAS (Wald $\chi^2 = z^2$). The p-values are the same, so the interpretation about the unique effect of the predictor variables is identical between the programs.

```
            (Dispersion parameter for binomial family taken to be 1)
Null deviance:              2241.5  on 1624  degrees of freedom
Residual deviance:          2220.9  on 1621  degrees of freedom
AIC:                        2228.9
Number of Fisher Scoring iterations: 4
```

Comment These are the values for model fit, and the null deviance matches the Intercept Only -2Loglikelihood in SAS, and the residual deviance is equivalent to the Intercepts and Covariates value. The AIC value here is the same as the AIC value for Intercepts and Covariates in the SAS output. The logistic regression model is best represented by

$$\log\left(\hat{P}_{biRadmit=1} / \hat{P}_{biRadmit=0}\right) = -0.2699 - 0.2903\text{DX}101 + 0.05799\text{NDX} + 0.0141\text{LOS}$$

```
> EXP(COEF(GLM.OUT))
Odds Ratio
(Intercept)             DX101           LOS          NDX
0.7634632           0.7480241       1.0142199     1.0597085
```

Comment These odds ratios are calculated by $e^{\text{maximumlikelihoodestimate}}$ where the maximum likelihood estimate is for the regression coefficient in the logit scale.

3.5.5 Analysis of Medicare Data with STATA Computing

Stata Program

```
STATA CODE
    . by time, sort: logistic biRadmit NDX    LOS DX101

Logistic regression           Number of obs =  1,625
                              LR chi2(3)    =  20.37
                              Prob > chi2   = 0.0001
Log likelihood = -1110.5668                  Pseudo R2      = 0.0091
  biRadmit  Coefficient  Std.err.   z      P>z  [95% conf.interval]
  NDX        .0582764    .0254343  2.29   0.022  .008426    .1081268
  LOS        .0141859    .0097461  1.46   0.146 -.0049162    .033288
  DX101     -.2826532    .1267257 -2.23   0.026 -.531031   -.0342753
  _cons     -.2736966    .1875397 -1.46   0.144 -.6412677   .0938746
```

Comment The estimate column contains the maximum likelihood estimates based on the logit scale. Note that the test statistics are z-scores. The confidence interval is given on the logit scale. The logistic regression model is best represented by

$$\log\left(\hat{P}_{biRadmit=1} / \hat{P}_{biRadmit=0}\right) = -0.2737 - 0.2826\text{DX101} + 0.0583\text{NDX} + 0.0142\text{LOS}$$

STATA CODE

```
.by time, sort : logistic biRadmit NDX    LOS DX101

Logistic regression          Number of obs =  1,625
             LR chi2(3)      = 20.37
             Prob > chi2     = 0.0001
     Log likelihood = -1110.5668          Pseudo R2      = 0.0091

biRadmit  Odds ratio  Std. err.    z      P>z  [95% conf. interval]
NDX        1.060008   .0269606    2.29   0.022  1.008462  1.114189
LOS        1.014287   .0098854    1.46   0.146   .9950958 1.033848
DX101      .7537812   .0955235   -2.23   0.026   .5879984 .9663054
_cons      .7605628   .1426358   -1.46   0.144   .5266244 1.098422
Note: _cons estimates baseline odds.
```

Comment The estimate column contains the maximum likelihood estimates for the odds ratio for that variable. For example, odds ratio of 1.06 (for NDX) tells if two patients had everything the same except one had an NDX 1 unit larger than the other and then the one with the larger NDX had an odd of 1.06 to get admit =1 versus admit = 0.

3.6 Conclusion

A standard logistic regression model with binary and continuous covariates can be very useful in a variety of situations. We modeled the probability of rehospitalization for patients within 30-days of discharge based on three predictors. The rehospitalization for each patient was considered a binary response. Through the standard logistic regression model, we were able to determine the odds of rehospitalization as related to the number of prescriptions, length of stay, and presence of coronary atherosclerosis. We were able to get a logistic regression model from which we could obtain predicted probabilities. However, we were careful with the characteristic values used for extrapolation and how they may have deviated from the present data. We were able to determine the number of procedures and whether or not certain diseases were important predictors of rehospitalization.

In future chapters, we will look at the larger dataset where patients were repeatedly observed regarding hospitalization and as such the data were correlated. In those cases, the standard logistic regression as presented in this chapter will not be appropriate.

3.7 Related Examples

Example 1 Consider the case where a banker is interested in the characteristics that determine whether a credit card should be issued to a customer. The outcome (response) variable is binary (0/1): whether a card should be issued (1) or do not issue a card (0). Some customer characteristics are income, age, amount of money spent on rent or mortgage, years of education, the number of late payments, and whether the customer has ever filed for bankruptcy. To answer this question, the banker can fit a logistic regression based on a sample of customer with the pertinent history. The fitted model can be used to determine the probability that the new customer should get a credit card.

Example 2 A school's associate dean for graduate programs is interested in variables such as GRE (graduate record exam) scores, undergraduate GPA (grade point average), and the prestige of the undergraduate institution which affect the admission into a graduate school program. He has 3 years of historical data on the success and failure of students admitted to a particular program. She will use a logistic regression model to present a model for admission. The outcome variable, admitted/not admitted, is binary (http://www.ats.ucla.edu/stat/sas/dae/logit.htm).

Questions

1. Describe why you would choose to analyze the graduate school data using a logistic regression as compared to a standard linear regression.
2. Using the maximum likelihood estimates from your output, describe the influence of GPA on the logit scale and on the probability of being accepted into graduate school.
3. Convert the maximum likelihood estimate and the upper and lower confidence limits of GPA into an odds ratio, and confirm your answer with the output.
4. Write one sentence that describes the influence of GPA on the odds of being accepted into graduate school.
5. Determine the influence of the institutions' prestige rankings on being accepted into graduate school by comparing the significance tests and confidence intervals.
6. Imagine you are giving a short speech to a high school class about the factors that influence acceptance into graduate school. Using the results from this example, write a short paragraph that describes what they should think about when applying for undergraduate programs to give them the best chance of being accepted into a graduate program in the future.

Appendix

Partial Medicare Data When Time = 1

PNUM_R	biRadmit	NDX	LOS	DX101	Time
127	0	9	6	1	1
560	1	9	8	0	1
746	1	6	12	0	1
750	0	9	6	0	1
1117	0	9	5	1	1
1395	1	9	6	0	1
1568	1	8	2	0	1
2076	1	9	8	1	1
2390	0	7	2	0	1
2413	0	9	17	0	1
3008	0	5	2	0	1
3123	1	9	3	0	1
3710	1	6	3	0	1
3970	0	9	1	0	1
3982	0	7	1	0	1
4236	0	9	5	0	1
4581	1	9	3	1	1
4873	0	9	1	1	1
5387	0	3	3	0	1
6255	0	9	5	0	1
7497	0	8	4	0	1
7599	0	7	4	1	1
8181	0	9	4	0	1
9677	1	2	1	1	1
10,464	0	8	4	0	1
11,050	0	4	1	0	1
11,274	0	9	13	0	1
14,955	0	8	3	0	1
16,160	0	2	0	0	1
16,464	1	9	4	0	1
16,971	0	8	8	0	1
17,748	0	9	3	0	1
18,638	0	9	6	0	1
18,697	1	7	3	0	1

References

Agresti, A. (2002). *Categorical data analysis* (2nd ed.). Wiley.

Akaike, H. (1981). Modern development of statistical methods. In P. Eykhoff (Ed.), *Trends and progress in system identification* (pp. 169–184). Pergamon Press.

Allison, P. D. (2008). Convergence failures in logistic regression. In *SAS Global Forum*, paper 360, pp. 1–11.

Allison, P. D. (2012). *Logistic regression using SAS: Theory and application* (2nd ed.). SAS Institute.

Cohen, J., Cohen, P., West, S. G., & Aiken, L. S. (2003). *Applied multiple regression/correlation analysis for the behavioral sciences* (3rd ed.). Erlbaum.

Cox, D. R., & Snell, E. J. (1989). *The analysis of binary data* (2nd ed.). Chapman & Hall.

Dobson, A. J., & Barnett, A. G. (2008). *An introduction to generalized linear models* (3rd ed.). Chapman & Hall.

Fang, D., Chong, J., & Wilson, J. R. (2015). Comparative predicted probabilities based on retrospective data with binary links. *American Journal of Public Health, 105*(5), 837–839.

Hosmer, D., & Lemeshow, W. (1989). *Applied logistic regression*. Wiley.

McCullagh, P., & Nelder, J. A. (1989). *Generalized linear models*. Chapman Hall.

McFadden, D. (1974). Conditional logit analysis of qualitative choice behavior. In P. Zarembka (Ed.), *Frontiers in econometrics*. Academic Press.

Nagelkerke, N. J. D. (1991). A note on a general definition of the coefficient of determination. *Biometrika, 78*(3), 691–692.

Nelder, J. A., & Wedderburn, R. W. M. (1972). Generalized linear models. *Journal of the Royal Statistical Society A, 135*(3), 370–384.

Oken, E., Kleinman, K. P., Belfort, M. B., Hammitt, J. K., & Gillman, M. W. (2009). Associations of gestational weight gain with short- and longer term maternal and child health outcomes. *American Journal of Epidemiology, 170*(2), 173–180.

Pregibon, D. (1981). Logistic regression diagnostics. *The Annals of Statistics, 9*(4), 705–724.

Simonoff, J. (2003). *Analyzing categorical data*. Springer.

Tjur, T. (2009). Coefficients of determination in logistic regression models – A new proposal: The coefficient of discrimination. *The American Statistician, 63*(4), 366–372.

Wang, S., & Carroll, R. J. (1999). High-order asymptotics for retrospective sampling problems. *Biometrika, 84*, 881–897.

Webb, M., Wilson, J. R., & Chong, J. (2004). An analysis of quasi-complete binary data withlogiticmodels: Applications to alcohol abuse data. *Journal of Data Science, 2*, 273–285.

Part II
Analyzing Correlated Data Through Random Component

Chapter 4
Overdispersed Logistic Regression Model

4.1 Motivating Example

A homeowner's association is interested in comparative housing satisfaction in two areas in a large city. The association wants to determine if the satisfaction of owners is somewhat related to whether or not they are living in a metropolitan city. At first glance, one may consider a simple analysis such as the Pearson's chi-square test and conduct a 2×2 analysis of satisfaction versus city or even a test of homogeneity depending on the sampling scheme. However, we learn that the data are not obtained from a simple random sample but rather in clusters (neighborhoods) from the metropolitan and nonmetropolitan city. The sampling scheme is not simple random sampling, and the clustering results in observations that are not independent. As such, the standard logistic regression model is not applicable. In particular, since the data were collected from households (clusters) and households tend to have common mechanism, it is doubtful to believe the outcomes were independently generated. Now that we are unable to use the standard logistic regression model, one wonders how to determine if the households in the metropolitan area have the same satisfaction level as those in the nonmetropolitan area. Recall that it is well known that the standard errors differ with clustering as opposed to obtaining the information based on a simple random sample. One wonders how the predictors impact the outcome as the data are based on clustering. Will the clustering result in less significant or more significant than if we had a simple random sample?

4.2 Definition and Notation

Since "overdispersion" is the key to the chapter, we provide a somewhat long discussion here with different expressions and definitions related to it.

J. R. Wilson et al., *Modeling Binary Correlated Responses*, ICSA Book Series in Statistics, https://doi.org/10.1007/978-3-031-62427-8_4

Overdispersion is a measure of the extent to which the clustered data are spread as compared to data consisting of independent observations. When binary data are obtained through simple random sampling, the covariance for the responses can be expected to satisfy the binomial sampling (two possible outcomes from independent observations with constant probability). However, when the data are obtained under cluster sampling, the covariance of the responses differs substantially from that of binomial. For example, clustering effects or subject effects in repeated measure experiments cause the variance of the observed proportions to be much larger than variance under the binomial assumption. The phenomenon is generally referred to as *overdispersion* or extra variation. The presence of overdispersion affects the standard errors and hence the conclusions made about significance of the predictors. The term *overdispersion* refers to the condition when the variance of an observed dependent (response) variable exceeds the nominal variance. This condition occurs frequently when fitting generalized linear models to correlated response data. Usually, the assumed distribution is binomial, multinomial, ordinal multinomial, or Poisson, wherever the variance and means are related. One does not talk about overdispersion in the so-called linear regression models as the variance is not related to the mean. When overdispersion occurs, the standard errors of the parameter estimates and related statistics (e.g., standard errors of predicted and residual statistics) are computed taking into account the overdispersion (Agresti, 2002); otherwise, you may incorrectly interpret test statistics. It is crucial to point out that there are various reasons for overdispersion. It may be due to outliers, misspecification of the model, variation between the response probabilities, or correlation between the binary outcomes.

Simple random sampling means that the researcher is using a subset of a 68
population in which each unit of the subset has an equal chance of being chosen. A simple random sample is meant to be an unbiased representation of the population. Consider an example of a simple random sample: A researcher chooses 200 households out of a metropolitan area which consists of 1000 households in total and out of a nonmetropolitan area which consists of 2000 households in total. Thus, there is simple random sample of 200 from a total of 3000. The sample is simple random because each household has an equal chance of being chosen. However, the sample may not be a good representation of the mixed population. A simple random sampling is more commonly used when the researcher knows little about the population, but if the researcher knew more, it would be better to use a different sampling technique. Schemes such as stratified random sampling, which helps to account for the differences (such as economic level or household size or age of head of household) within the population, require more information.

4.3 Exploratory Data Analyses

In the household satisfaction survey, the response (satisfied versus unsatisfied) versus area (metropolitan versus nonmetropolitan) results in a 2×2 classification as presented in Table 4.1.

Table 4.1 Cross-classification of response by city

Response	Nonmetropolitan = 0	Metropolitan = 1
Unsatisfied	47	30
Satisfied	43	55

The odds ratio is 3.68 (p = 0.0241), which suggests that homeowners in nonmetropolitan areas = 0 were 3.68 times more likely to be unsatisfied than homeowners living in the metropolitan area = 1. The data in Table 4.1 are based on results of the clustering or grouping received for each of the 35 clusters (18 from nonmetropolitan =0 and 17 from metropolitan = 1). Any differential effects due to the neighborhoods were ignored. By ignoring any such effects, one is in fact saying that the neighborhoods effects are all the same. This is dangerous because ignoring the clustering or overdispersion leads to incorrect standard errors. The presence of overdispersion denies us the opportunity to have a joint likelihood of the 175 observations, as we do not have independent observations.

This chapter presents a method of analyzing binary grouped data in the presence of overdispersion. The assumed distribution of the sample proportion is not known, but it is assumed that the variance and covariance are functions of the population proportions with a limited number of scaling parameters. Parameter estimates are obtained through a combination of generalized least squares, and moment estimation techniques and large sample chi-square tests are developed. Our model in Fig. 4.1 allows any kinds of covariate (binary, categorical, or continuous) as input. The output is binary. However, each outcome is not independent of the other.

If we used the standard logistic regression to model these data, then the model variance is smaller to what is really in the data. This phenomenon as we have stated is known as overdispersion, because the true model variance is greater than expected. It allows us to conclude that things are significant when in fact they are not. Such is the case in the household satisfaction survey analyzed in Sect. 4.5.

4.4 Statistical Model

It has often been observed that variances of sample proportions exceed those implied by Poisson, binomial, or multinomial distributions. This *variance discrepancy*, Ehrenberg (1959), limits the direct applicability of models involving these distributions. In these cases, the sample proportions are often referred to as being overdispersed. Efron (1986) suggested that such a phenomenon may be caused by clumped sampling. Cox (1983) points out that overdispersion in general has two effects:

1. Summary statistics from the clustered data have a larger variance than anticipated under the simple model (so, if ignored, one can say that something is significant when in fact it is not).
2. There is a possible loss of efficiency when using statistics that are appropriate for the single-parameter family. The independent binomial is a member of a single-

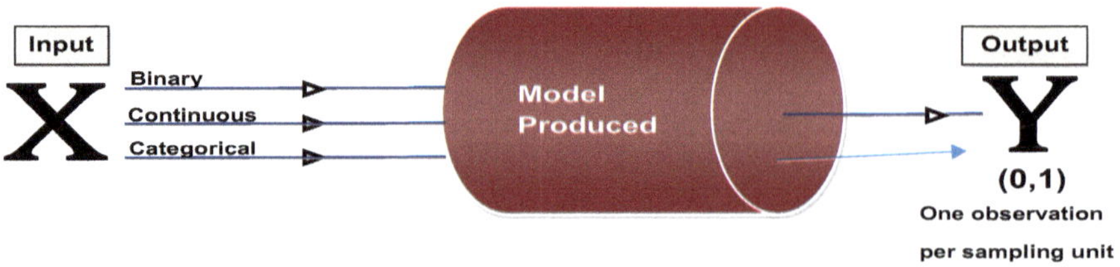

Fig. 4.1 Schematic diagram of **X** impacting **Y**

parameter family, but the overdispersed binomial model introduces a second parameter through the overdispersion factor.

There are three basic approaches (Wilson & Koehler, 1991) to solving problems with such overdispersed data:

1. The first approach depends on constructing appropriate quadratic forms, usually seen as Wald statistics. This approach relies on the properties of the sampling distribution of the observed vectors of frequencies.
2. A second approach is to accept that while the distribution of the observations may be difficult or impossible to detect, the form of the mean-variance relationship is often much easier to present. This technique is a type of method of moment approach, as it relies only on the form of the mean and variance. This approach is common (Altham, 1978; Williams, 1982). Similarly, Bartlett (1937) presented $var(y_i) = \phi^2\mu(1 + a\mu)$ for counts from field trials, while Armitage (1957) found that in the variability of pock counts $var(y_i) = \phi^2\mu^b$ with $1 < b < 2$ to be useful, and for the most part $\phi^2 > 1$. Another, similar approach is the quasi-likelihood (Wedderburn (1974), McCullagh (1983), and Wilson (1989)). These methods rely on the asymptotic properties of the estimators (Moore, 1986).
3. Another approach is to allow the distributions to have an additional parameter to account for the overdispersion. This results in the generalization of the distribution. Examples include the beta-binomial (Williams, 1975; Crowder, 1978; Chatfield & Goodhart, 1970) and the Dirichlet-multinomial models (Brier, 1980; Koehler & Wilson, 1986). Crowder investigated the extra variation in the regression analysis of proportions. Brier (1980) and Koehler and Wilson (1986) presented models based on the use of the Dirichlet-multinomial models. The models are referred to as constant design effects models (Rao and Scott (1981)). Rao and Scott provided an approximate method of rescaling chi-square tests to adjust for the effects of overdispersion arising from complex sample surveys. Bedrick (1983) used partial information about the covariance matrix of the observed vector of frequencies to make adjustment to test statistics for log-linear models. McCullagh and Nelder (1989) presented examples for which extra variation is modeled by multiplying the covariance matrix for a vector of binomial, Poisson, or multinomial proportions by a single scaling factor. The advantage of these distributional assumptions is the parameters may be estimated by maximum likelihood. Maximum likelihood estimators are known to be consistent, asymptotically normally distributed, and efficient (Moore (1986)). In addition, Pack

(1986) found that likelihood ratio tests (these are based on maximum likelihood estimators) are at least as powerful as the simpler approaches and in certain situations can be significantly more powerful.

In this chapter, we fit overdispersed logistic regression models based on Williams' method and an exchangeable logistic regression model to the grouped data. Both models provide an accounting of the overdispersion through the variance and covariance. One model applies a factor to the variance under independent observations, while the latter model applies a common correlation between any two observations. They give similar results.

4.4.1 Williams' Method of Analysis

Consider m neighborhoods, and within each neighborhood (cluster), we measure each unit or a sample of units and take note of a binary outcome. We fit a logistic regression model to the correlated binomial responses. The correlation is inherent due to the clustering effect, meaning responses within a neighborhood would tend to be more similar to each other than expected from a simple random sample. On account of this clustering, we cannot use maximum likelihood since the joint distribution of the responses is not fully specified. We cannot take the product of the individual probabilities to create a likelihood function when data are correlated. However, we specify a mean-variance relationship and apply a quasi-likelihood approach to account for overdispersion. In fact, we postulate that the probability of success is the same within the cluster but differs across clusters. Thus, we present a two-level nested logistic regression model in which the top-level response is binomially distributed, conditional on the probability of success (Williams, 1982). This probability of success varies across clusters and as such has an unknown distribution. We assume that we have a known mean-variance relationship that accounts for overdispersion through a multiplicative factor.

The model (Williams, 1982) assumes that the response Y_i in level 1 is binomially distributed conditional on the probability p_i such that

$$Y_i | p_i \sim Bin(m_i, p_i)$$

where m_i is the total sample size at cluster i. At level 2, we have a distribution (though unknown) of the probabilities such that

$$p_i \sim Dist_{p_i}\left(\theta_i, \sigma_{p_i}^2\right)$$

where

$$\sigma_{p_i}^2 = \varphi\theta_i\left(1-\theta_i\right),$$

suggesting

$$\text{Variance} = \{\text{factor}\}\,\text{times}\left[\text{function of the mean}\right]$$

$0 < \theta_i < 1$ is an unknown parameter, $\varphi > 0$ is the overdispersion factor, and $Dist_{p_i}$ denotes the distribution of p_i. The distribution $Dist_{p_i}$ is still unknown, but the mean-variance relationship is known up to the parameter φ. Once this parameter is estimated, we can fit the overdispersion logistic regression model. The overdispersion factor sometimes referred to as the heterogeneity factor inflates the elements of the covariance matrix of the parameter estimates. One way to estimate the overdispersion factor is to use the ratio of Pearson or deviance statistic to its degrees of freedom. The model assumes the relationship

$$\log\left(\frac{P(Y=1)}{P(Y=0)}\right) = \beta_0 X_0 + \beta_1 X_1 + \ldots\ldots\beta_p X_p$$

with variance factored by a constant. We fit such models using PROC GENMOD in SAS and R. One can also fit such overdispersed models using the generalized estimating equations (GEE) method (Morel & Neerchal, 1997) as shown in Chap. 6.

4.4.2 Overdispersion Factor

In practice, if an estimate of the overdispersion factor after fitting (i.e., as measured by the deviance or Pearson's chi-square, divided by the degrees of freedom) is not near one, then the data might be *overdispersed* (if the overdispersion factor is greater than one) or *underdispersed* (if the overdispersion factor is less than one). It is useful to note that an overdispersion factor of significance might also indicate other problems such as an incorrectly specified model or outliers in the data. Thus, one needs to carefully assess whether this type of model is appropriate for your data. While an approach to obtain the overdispersion factor is to take the ratio of the goodness-of-fit statistics to the degrees of freedom, applying this adjustment causes other issues. Obtaining the function obtained by dividing a log-likelihood function for the binomial or Poisson distribution by a dispersion parameter is not a legitimate log-likelihood function. In fact, it is considered a quasi-likelihood function. However, the asymptotic theory for log likelihoods applies to quasi-likelihoods, which justifies computing standard errors and likelihood ratio statistics by using quasi-likelihoods instead of proper log likelihoods (Hardin & Hilbe, 2003; McCullagh & Nelder, 1989; Chap. 9).

4.4.3 *Datasets*

In this chapter, we present two datasets, *Housing Satisfaction Survey* and *Use of Word Einai*. We will analyze the first example in Sect. 4.6 and provide the readers with a second example to help them use the overdispersed model.

4.4.4 *Housing Satisfaction Survey*

A study of housing satisfaction was conducted to analyze their degree of satisfaction homeowners felt based on their type of living conditions (Brier, 1980). These data were obtained on the basis of a stratified two-stage cluster sampling scheme. The variance of sample proportions for the categories of satisfaction is expected to be overdispersed. Thus, different weights are associated with the categories of the vector of proportions from different strata. This seems to be a clear case when overdispersion may be present if we used the standard logistic regression model.

4.5 Analysis of Data

In this chapter, we will revisit data from a study of housing satisfaction performed by H. S. Stoeckler and M. G. Gate for the US Department of Agriculture (Brier, 1980). Households around Montevideo, Minnesota, were stratified into two populations: those in the metropolitan area and those outside the metropolitan area. A random sample of 20 neighborhoods was taken from each population, and 5 households were randomly selected from each of the sampled neighborhoods. One response was obtained from the residents of each household concerning their satisfaction with their home. The possible responses were "unsatisfied" (US), "satisfied" (S), and "very satisfied" (VS). However, for our analysis, we did (Koehler & Wilson, 1986) a binary variable of US versus S and VS. Only data from neighborhoods in which responses were obtained from each of the five households sampled were used to illustrate the usefulness of the model. Thus, the dataset contains $K_1 = 18$ neighborhoods from the nonmetropolitan area and $K_2 = 17$ neighborhoods from the metropolitan area. We fit a logistic regression model to a binary response of unsatisfied versus satisfied with area as a covariate. The data (Table 4.2) are given in grouped form rather than ungrouped (where each row corresponds to an individual measure). The COUNT represents the number of satisfied homeowners in each neighborhood, and as such, the data are considered grouped. The TOTAL is the cluster size. We fit the standard logistic and then the overdispersed logistic regression using PROC GENMOD in SAS and R. We also fit the exchangeable logistic regression model.

Table 4.2 Housing satisfaction survey by city and neighborhood

Metro	nghbd	Count	Total	Metro	nghbd	Count	Total
0	1	2	5	1	1	5	5
0	2	2	5	1	2	5	5
0	3	5	5	1	3	5	5
0	4	2	5	1	4	2	5
0	5	5	5	1	5	3	5
0	6	1	5	1	6	4	5
0	7	2	5	1	7	1	5
0	8	3	5	1	8	1	5
0	9	1	5	1	9	5	5
0	10	5	5	1	10	4	5
0	11	3	5	1	11	5	5
0	12	1	5	1	12	2	5
0	13	1	5	1	13	3	5
0	14	4	5	1	14	3	5
0	15	1	5	1	15	1	5
0	16	4	5	1	16	5	5
0	17	1	5	1	17	1	5
0	18	0	5				

4.5.1 *Standard Logistic Regression Model*

We fitted the standard logistic model in Chap. 3, and in this chapter, we are going to revisit application to Brier's data for completeness in our comparisons. Since Chap. 3 provides all the details for a standard logistic regression model using SAS and R, we only presented results from SAS.

SAS Program

```
DATA brier19801;
set Brier1980;
PROC LOGISTIC DATA=brier19801;
MODEL count/total=metro/SCALE=NONE;
TITLE 'FULL MODEL WITH SCALE=NONE'; RUN;
```

Comment PROC LOGISTIC is used to fit a standard logistic regression model to the data, with metropolitan area *{rural* versus *urban}* as a covariate. There is an option "scale" in this procedure that was used to display goodness-of-fit statistics. This model with "SCALE = NONE" ignores the clustering inherent in the neighborhoods.

SAS Output

The logistic procedure	
Model information	
Dataset	WORK.BRIER19801
Response variable (events)	Count
Response variable (trials)	Total
Model	Binary logit
Optimization technique	Fisher's scoring
Number of observations read	35
Number of observations used	35
Sum of frequencies read	175
Sum of frequencies used	175

Comment The number of observations read is the number of clusters corresponding to the primary sampling units. The frequencies read of 35 × 5 = 175 are the total number of observational or secondary units. The data are grouped.

Response profile		
Ordered value	Binary outcome	Total frequency
1	Event	98
2	Nonevent	77

Model convergence status				
Convergence criterion (GCONV = 1E-8) satisfied				
Deviance and Pearson goodness-of-fit statistics				
Criterion	Value	DF	Value/DF	Pr > ChiSq
Deviance	90.8733	33	2.7537	<0.0001
Pearson	73.2012	33	2.2182	<0.0001

Comment Results of fitting the model indicate a poor fit. Both Pearson statistic = 73.20 and deviance statistics = 90.87 are highly significant ($p < 0.0001$) suggesting that the model does not fit. It is possible that the lack-of-fit is due to overdispersion. As we pointed out, the cause of that overdispersion is multifold. It depends on whether the link function {i.e., link between probability and the covariate, in this case the logit} and the model specification are correct and if there are no outliers. We will assume that we have the correct model specification and correct link function. If we do not adjust for the overdispersion, the standard errors we assumed based on the binomial assumption are likely to be smaller than their true value. Thus, if there is correlation and it is ignored, then the statistical tests are too sensitive. Thus, the test may give significance and it is not.

SAS Output

Model fit statistics			
Criterion	Intercept only	Intercept and covariates	With constant
AIC	242.075	238.961	143.240
SC	245.240	245.290	149.569
−2 Log L	240.075	234.961	139.240

Testing global null hypothesis: BETA = 0			
Test	Chi-square	DF	Pr > ChiSq
Likelihood ratio	5.1146	1	0.0237
Score	5.0839	1	0.0241
Wald	5.0300	1	0.0249

Comment The test for the effect of the covariate is significant. The goodness-of-fit tests for the standard logistic regression model were all based on the assumption that the satisfaction within each of the neighborhoods was independent Bernoulli trials (and the trials across neighborhoods were independent).

Analysis of maximum likelihood estimates					
Parameter	DF	Estimate	Standard error	Wald Chi-square	Pr > ChiSq
Intercept	1	−0.0889	0.2110	0.1777	0.6734
Metro	1	0.6951	0.3099	5.0300	0.0249

Comment Under this within-neighborhood independence assumption, we rejected the standard logistic regression model. However, in the standard logistic regression model, within-neighborhood independent trial assumption is unreasonable, and the goodness-of-fit tests are of questionable validity. The standard error is 0.3099 corresponding to the variation among estimate for metropolitan area versus nonmetropolitan area {of significance ($p = 0.0249$)} is also of questionable validity, as its computation used the independence assumption. Thus, we reject the model of

$$\log\left\{\frac{p_s}{p_{us}}\right\} = -0.0889 + 0.6951\,Metro$$

As such, we do not interpret the odds ratio of [1.092, 3.678]. The standard error for metro is 0.3099.

Odds ratio estimates			
Effect	Point estimate	95% Wald confidence limits	
Metro	2.004	1.092	3.678

Association of predicted probabilities and observed responses			
Percent concordant	34.3	Somers' D	0.172
Percent discordant	17.1	Gamma	0.334
Percent tied	48.6	Tau-A	0.085
Pairs	7546	c	0.586

Comment The fact that the standard logistic regression probability model was rejected (using the independence assumption) could be due to at least two reasons:

1. The common probability assumption across the neighborhoods within city is in fact not true.
2. The common probability assumption across the neighborhoods could be true, but the independence assumption is not; if there is positive within-neighborhood correlation, we would expect overdispersion.

4.5.2 Overdispersed Logistic Regression Model

Though the metropolitan area showed a significant impact on satisfaction, one cannot interpret, as the model does not fit. Instead, we address the overdispersion and then fitted the overdispersed logistic regression model. We modeled the potential overdispersion through the binomial assumption and use the semi-parametric (quasibinomial) model:

$$Y_i \mid household_i \sim Bin\left(n_i, p_{household_i}\right)$$

$$p_{household_i} \sim Dist_{unknown_i}\left(\pi_i, \varphi\pi_i\left(1-\pi_i\right)\right)$$

So, the unconditional distribution of Y_i is not fully known, but the mean-variance relation is $var\ (Y_i) = \varphi n_i \pi_i (1 - \pi_i)$. Here, y_i is the number of satisfied households i, $i = 1, 2, \ldots, n_j$; and $j = 1, 2$; represents the two areas. To fit this model, we used PROC LOGISTIC with option scale = Williams.

4.5.3 *Overdispersed Logistic Regression Model Using SAS Program*

SAS Program

```
PROC LOGISTIC DATA=brier19801;
MODEL count/total=metro/SCALE=WILLIAMS;
TITLE 'OVERDISPERSION MODEL WITH SCALE=WILLIAMS';
RUN;
```

Comment The SCALE = option in the MODEL statement enables you to specify a value of $\sigma = \sqrt{\varphi}$ for the binomial and Poisson distributions. If you specify the SCALE = DEVIANCE option in the MODEL statement, the procedure uses the deviance divided by degrees of freedom as an estimate of φ, and all statistics are adjusted appropriately. You can use Pearson's chi-square instead of the deviance by specifying the SCALE = PEARSON option.

SAS Output

Overdispersion model with scale = WILLIAMS	
The logistic procedure	
Model information	
Dataset	WORK.BRIER19801
Response variable (events)	Count
Response variable (trials)	Total
Weight variable	1/(1 + 0.304556 * (Total – 1))
Model	Binary logit
Optimization technique	Fisher's scoring

Comment The overdispersion factor is estimated to be 0.3046.

Number of observations read	35
Number of observations used	35
Sum of frequencies read	175
Sum of frequencies used	175
Sum of weights read (44.18 + 34.71) =	78.89191
Sum of weights used	78.89191

Response profile			
Ordered value	**Binary outcome**	**Total frequency**	**Total weight**
1	Event	98	44.179470
2	Nonevent	77	34.712441

Comment The weights changed from 98:77 in standard logistic regression model to 44.18:34.71. An estimate of φ is 0.3046 and is given in the formula for the weight variable. If $\varphi = 0$ then the weight variable is 1. If $\varphi = 1$ then the weight variable is 1/total.

Model convergence status
Convergence criterion (GCONV = 1E-8) satisfied

Deviance and Pearson goodness-of-fit statistics				
Criterion	**Value**	**DF**	**Value/DF**	**Pr > ChiSq**
Deviance	40.9667	33	1.2414	0.1606
Pearson	32.9999	33	1.0000	0.4673

Comment Based on the value/DF, we are inclined to say that the model fits. Since the Williams' method was used to accommodate overdispersion, the Pearson's chi-square statistic and the deviance can no longer be used to assess the goodness-of-fit of the model. Therefore, we must rely on the other fit indices to compare the relative fit of the model accounting for overdispersion. However, the metropolitan city is not statistically significant (p = 0.1321).

Number of events/trials observations: 35

Model fit statistics			
Criterion	**Intercept only**	**Intercept and covariates**	**With constant**
AIC	110.229	109.923	66.771
SC	113.393	116.253	73.100
−2 Log L	108.229	105.923	62.771

Testing global null hypothesis: Beta = 0			
Test	**Chi-square**	**DF**	**Pr > ChiSq**
Likelihood ratio	2.3057	1	0.1289
Score	2.2919	1	0.1301
Wald	2.2676	1	0.1321

Analysis of maximum likelihood estimates					
Parameter	**DF**	**Estimate**	**Standard error**	**Wald chi-square**	**Pr > ChiS**
Intercept	1	−0.0889	0.3143	0.0801	0.7772
Metro	1	0.6951	0.4616	2.2676	0.1321

Comment The estimates are the same as in the standard logistic regression, but the standard errors are changed. It was 0.3099 and it is now 0.4616. There is a multiplicative factor of 1.4895 = 0.4616/0.3099 for the standard errors and 2.2182 = 1.4895^2 for the variance.

$$\log\left\{\frac{p_s}{p_{us}}\right\} = -0.0889 + 0.6951\,Metro$$

Odds ratio estimates			
Effect	**Point estimate**	**95% Wald confidence limits**	
Metro	2.004	0.811	4.952

Association of predicted probabilities and observed responses			
Percent concordant	34.3	Somers' D	0.172
Percent discordant	17.1	Gamma	0.334
Percent tied	48.6	Tau-a	0.085
Pairs	7546	c	0.586

Comment The estimates of the logit and odds ratio do not change (still equal to 0.6951), but their standard errors do change. The results showed that once we have adjusted for the overdispersion, the perceived difference between metropolitan and nonmetropolitan areas is no longer significant (p = 0.1321). Results of using Williams' methodology shows that an estimate of φ is 0.3046 and is given in the formula for the weight variable at the beginning of the displayed output. The overdispersion factor is included in the weight variable with the observations weighted by [1/(1 + 0.3046(N − 1))] that are the scaling factor matrix for the standard errors. If there was within-neighborhood correlation among the neighborhoods, it would most likely be of a positive nature; either the neighborhood is satisfied or not. The within-neighborhood positive correlation will tend to result in more neighborhood-to-neighborhood variability in the proportion of satisfied households than would be expected if the within-neighborhood satisfaction were independent. So the within-neighborhood correlation leads to more similar responses within that cluster, and therefore when examining between neighborhoods, there is a greater variation in expected values of satisfaction scores. Since we are modeling between-neighborhood influences, the clustering within a neighborhood introduces an extra source of variation that we are not accounting for under the assumption of independence. That is, within-neighborhood positive correlation will likely lead to *overdispersion* relative to what is expected in the binomial model that assumes independence.

4.5.4 Overdispersed Logistic Regression Model Using R Program

R Program

```
Call:
glm(formula = count/total ~ Metro, family = quasibinomial(logit),
data = data1)
```

Comment This is the code for running the model in R. We need the quasibinomial.

R Output

Deviance Residuals:

Min	1Q	Median	3Q	Max
-1.13988	-0.57801	-0.09758	0.79852	1.21541

Comment The residuals are given as they give insight into the fit of the model. The residuals lie within [−1.140, 1.215].

Coefficients:

	Estimate	Std. Error	t value	Pr(>|t|)
(Intercept)	-0.08895	0.31430	-0.283	0.779
Metro	0.69508	0.46158	1.506	0.142

Comment The estimates are the same as in the standard logistic regression, but the standard errors are changed. It was 0.3099 and it is now 0.4616. There is a multiplicative factor of 1.4895 = 0.4616/0.3099 for the standard errors and $2.2182 = 1.4895^2$ for the variance.

$$\log\left\{\frac{p_s}{p_{us}}\right\} = -0.0889 + 0.6951\,Metro$$

(Dispersion parameter for quasibinomial family taken to be 0.4436451)
Null deviance: 19.198 on 34 degrees of freedom.
Residual deviance: 18.175 on 33 degrees of freedom.
AIC: NA.
Number of Fisher's scoring iterations: 3.

Comment Based on the value/DF, we are inclined to say that the model fits. Since the Williams' method was used to accommodate overdispersion, the Pearson's chi-square statistic and the deviance can no longer be used to assess the goodness-of-fit of the model. Therefore, we must rely on the other fit indices to compare the relative fit of the model accounting for overdispersion. However, the metropolitan city is not statistically significant (p = 0.142).

4.5.5 Exchangeability Logistic Regression Model

In similar fashion, we fitted an exchangeable logistic regression model. In this model, we assumed that the correlation between any two units is the same. We fitted the model with SAS and R.

4.5.6 Exchangeability Logistic Regression Model Using SAS Program

SAS Program

```
PROC GENMOD DATA=BRIER19801 DESC;
CLASS NGHBD;
  MODEL COUNT/TOTAL=METRO/dist=binomial link=logit
aggregate=(NGHBD) scale=p;
  REPEATED SUBJECT=NGHBD/TYPE= EXCH;
RUN;
```

Comment We fitted a model where we assumed that the correlation is the same in each neighborhood within each area. This is essentially the compound symmetry or exchangeable model in generalized estimating equations. We computed this in SAS with PROC GENMOD and TYPE = EXCH (invoking the common correlation assumption). The advantage of using compound symmetry/exchangeability assumption, which may not always be practical, is the fact that we only have one extra parameter to estimate.

SAS Output

The GENMOD procedure	
Model information	
Dataset	WORK.BRIER19801
Distribution	Binomial
Link function	Logit
Response variable (events)	Count
Response variable (trials)	Total
Number of observations read	35
Number of observations used	35
Number of events	98
Number of trials	175

Comment The number read refers to the clusters. The data were presented in group form. There are 175 units of which 98 units are satisfied.

Class level information		
Class	Levels	Values
nghbd	18	1 2 3 4 5 6 7 8 9 10 11 12 13 14 15 16 17 18

Comment There are 18 clusters listed although there are 17 and 18 in the two cities. It lists the larger of the number of clusters.

Response profile		
Ordered value	Binary outcome	Total frequency
1	Event	98
2	Nonevent	77

Parameter information	
Parameter	Effect
Prm1	Intercept
Prm2	Metro

Algorithm converged	
GEE model information	
Correlation structure	Exchangeable
Subject effect	nghbd (18 levels)
Number of clusters	18
Correlation matrix dimension	2
Maximum cluster size	2
Minimum cluster size	1

Algorithm converged	
Exchangeable working correlation	
Correlation	0.3270

Comment In the Williams' model, we had a factor of 0.3046 as opposed to 0.3270 in the exchangeability model. Although we present clusters of size 5, we see a correlation matrix dimension of 2.

Analysis of GEE parameter estimates						
Empirical standard error estimates						
Parameter	Estimate	Standard error	95% confidence limits		Z	Pr > |Z|
Intercept	−0.0889	0.2963	−0.6697	0.4918	−0.30	0.7640
Metro	0.6566	0.3691	−0.0669	1.3801	1.78	0.0753

Comment The common correlation model is estimated to have a value of $r_{period_i period_j} = 0.3270$ that is used to compute the overdispersion factor, and as this correlation approaches 1.0, overdispersion poses a serious problem in the analysis and must be addressed. The overdispersion factor in the Williams' model was $\hat{\varphi} = 0.3046$. The exchangeable model also reported whether or not the neighborhood was in a metropolitan or a nonmetropolitan area. The model is

$$\log\left\{\frac{p_s}{p_{us}}\right\} = -0.0889 + 0.6566\,Metro$$

Model information			
Events variable		Count	
Trials variable		Total	
Probability distribution		Binomial	
Link function		Logit	
Subject effect	1	nghbd	
Working correlation matrix structure		Exchangeable	
Case processing summary			
	N	Percent (%)	
Included	35	100.0	
Excluded	0	0.0	
Total	35	100.0	
Correlated data summary			
Number of levels	Subject effect	nghbd	18
Number of subjects			18
Number of measurements per subject	Minimum		1
	Maximum		2
Correlation matrix dimension			2

Categorical variable information				
			N	Percent (%)
Dependent variable[a]	Count	Events	98	56.0
		Nonevents	77	44.0
		Total	175	100.0

[a]Trials variable: total

Continuous variable information						
		N	Minimum	Maximum	Mean	Std. deviation
Covariate	Metro	35	0	1	0.49	0.507

Goodness-of-fit[a]	
	Value
Quasi-likelihood under Independence Model Criterion (QIC)[b]	462.804
Corrected quasi-likelihood under Independence Model Criterion (QICC)[b]	458.511
Events: Count; trials: Total; model: (intercept), Metro[a]	

[a]Information criteria are in small-is-better form
[b]Computed using the full log quasi-likelihood function

Tests of model effects			
Source	Type III		
	Wald chi-square	DF	Sig.
(Intercept)	0.090	1	0.764
Metro	3.164	1	0.075
Events: Count; trials: Total; model: (intercept), metro			

4.5.7 *Exchangeability Logistic Regression Model Using R Program*

R Program

```
GEEGLM (with repeated subject=nghbd and correlation type =exchange)
Call:
geeglm(formula = count/total ~ Metro, family = binomial(logit),
 data = data1, id = nghbd, corstr = "exchangeable")
```

Comment the R code for the exchangeable logistic regression model.

R Output

```
Coefficients:
                Estimate     Std.err       Wald        Pr(>|W|)
(Intercept)    -0.08895      0.29633       0.090       0.764
Metro           0.69508      0.44953       2.391       0.122
```

Comment The fitted logistic regression model is

$$log\left\{\frac{p_s}{p_{us}}\right\} = -0.0889 + 0.6951\,Metro.$$

Metro is not significant in the model in explaining household satisfaction.

```
Estimated Scale Parameters:
                      Estimate        Std.err
(Intercept)            0.4183         0.06529
```

Comment A measure of the correlation or overdispersion is measured as 0.4183. There is a standard error of 0.06529. A test suggests that (0.4183/0.06529) = 6.41 is significant.

```
Correlation: Structure = exchangeable Link = identity
Estimated Correlation Parameters:
             Estimate    Std.err
alpha            0              0
Number of clusters:   35   Maximum cluster size: 1
```

Comment Metro is not significant in the model.

4.6 Conclusion

Routine use of the standard logistic regression model in the presence of any kind of complex sampling schemes should be avoided. The assumption of independence, thereby ignoring the overdispersion, seriously underestimates the standard errors for the regression coefficients. One possible approach is to assume the GEE model with compound symmetry as the covariance structure or another approach to use Williams' overdispersed logistic regression which adjusts for the extra variation. In our example, metropolitan area was no longer a significant factor once we adjusted for the extra variation. The response to satisfaction with their homes seems to be consistent whether they were in the metropolitan or nonmetropolitan area. We used SAS and R to analyze the data.

Both the overdispersed logistic regression model and the exchangeable logistic regression model use adjustments to the covariance matrix to account for the clustering which leads to correlation and overdispersion. The difference in these models is minimal. One model assumes that all relationships are assumed to be the same, and the adjustment is to factor up the standard error from independent observations. The second model also allows a common relationship. It corrects for it through the construction at the early stage. Thus, the covariance matrix provides slight difference numerically in the standard error. One model assumes the adjustment was a single factor, while the other model assumes the relationship between any two units within the cluster.

4.7 Related Example

4.7.1 Use of Word Einai

Overdispersed data, concerning the use of the word *einai* (*einai* is the Greek word meaning "to be"), are presented in Morton (1965). Books were randomly sampled from each of the works of two Greek authors, Thucydides and Herodotus. The occurrences of *einai* in the chosen sentences within each book were categorized according to the number of *einai* (no *einai*, one *einai*, two *einai*, three *einai*, or greater than three *einai*). The sample vectors of proportions are expected to be overdispersed with different weights associated with each category. We consider the books as clusters. These data are provided in http://www.public.asu.edu/~jeffreyw.

Some relevant questions

1. Suppose the researcher wants to know if the use of *einai* (used or not used) differs between the two Greek authors and uses a standard logistic regression, what will be his/her conclusions?
2. Suppose you were told that the rate of occurrences differs across books, what will you do to analyze the data while taking into consideration the added information?
3. Do you have any evidence that the data are overdispersed?

References

Agresti, A. (2002). *Categorical data analysis* (2nd ed.). Wiley.

Altham, P. M. E. (1978). Two generalizations of the binomial distribution. *Journal of the Royal Statistical Society Series C, Royal Statistical Society, 27*(2), 162–167.

Armitage, P. (1957). Studies in the variability of pock counts. *Epidemiology & Infection, 55*(4), 564–581.

Bartlett, M. S. (1937). The statistical conception of mental factors. *British journal of Psychology, 28*(1), 97.
Bedrick, E. J. (1983). Adjusted goodness-of-fit tests for survey data. *Biometrika, 70*, 591.
Brier, S. S. (1980). Analysis of contingency tables under cluster sampling. *Biometrika, 67*, 591–596.
Chatfield, C., & Goodhart, G. J. (1970). The beta-binomial model for consumer purchasing behaviour. *Applied Statistics, 19*, 240–250.
Cox, D. R. (1983). Some remarks on overdispersion. *Biometrika, 70*, 269–274.
Crowder, M. J. (1978). Beta-binomial ANOVA for proportions. *Applied Statistics, 27*, 34–37.
Efron, B. E. (1986). Double exponential families and their use in generalized linear regression. *Journal of the American Statistical Association, 81*, 709–721.
Ehrenberg, A. S. C. (1959). The Pattern of Consumer Purchases. *Journal of the Royal Statistical Society Series C (Applied Statistics), 8*(1), 26–41. https://doi.org/10.2307/2985810
Hardin, J., & Hilbe, J. (2003). *Generalized estimating equations*. Chapman and Hall.
Koehler, K. J., & Wilson, J. R. (1986). Chi-square tests for comparing vectors of proportions for several cluster samples. *Communications in Statistics: Theory and Methods, 15*, 2977–2990.
McCullagh , P. (1983) Quasi-likelihood functions. *Ann Statist, 11*, 59–67.
McCullagh, P., & Nelder, J. A. (1989). *Generalized linear models* (2nd ed.). Chapman and Hall.
Moore, D. F. (1986). Asymptotic properties of moment estimators for overdispersed counts and proportions. *Biometrika, 73*, 583–588.
Morel, J. G., & Neerchal, N. K. (1997). Clustered binary logistic regression in teratology data using a finite mixture distribution. *Statistics in Medicine, 16*, 2843–2853.
Morton, A. Q. (1965). The authorship of Greek prose (with discussion). *Journal of the Royal Statistical Society A, 128*, 169–233.
Pack, S. E. (1986). Hypothesis testing for proportions with overdispersion. *Biometrics, 42*, 967–972.
Rao, J. N. K., & Scott, A. J. (1981). The analysis of categorical data from complex surveys. *Journal of the American Statistical Association, 76*, 221–230.
Wedderburn, R. W. M. (1974). Quasi-likelihood functions, generalised linear models, and the gauss-Newton method. *Biometrika, 61*, 439–447.
Williams, D. A. (1975). The analysis of binary responses from toxicological experiments involving reproduction and heterogeneity. *Biometrics, 31*, 949–952.
Williams, D. A. (1982). Extra-binomial variation in logistic linear models. *Applied Statistics, 31*, 144–148.
Wilson, J. R. (1989). Chi-square tests for overdispersion with multiparameter estimates. *Journal of Royal Statistics Society Series C, Applied Statistics, 38*(3), 441–454.
Wilson, J. R., & Koehler, K. J. (1991). Hierarchical models for cross-classified overdispersed multinomial data. *Journal of Business and Economic Statistics, 9*(1), 103–110.

Chapter 5
Weighted Logistic Regression Model

5.1 Motivating Example

It is common to have binary responses in surveys (e.g., yes/no, agree/disagree, purchased/not purchased). These responses are modeled through binary models, a relationship between the probability of that response and a set of covariates. However, as we saw in Chap. 4, when the data are not obtained by simple random sampling, the standard logistic regression is not valid. When binary data are obtained from clusters of different sizes, we used an overdispersion factor to adjust the variance, as discussed in Chap. 4. However, in this chapter, we present a more efficient method than using a common dispersion factor adjustment.

When data come from a complex survey design with stratification, clustering, and/or unequal weighting, the usual estimates are not appropriate (Rao & Scott, 1984). In these cases, specialized techniques must be applied in order to produce reliable and consistent estimates for their standard errors. In Chap. 4, we used the overdispersed logistic regression and exchangeability logistic regression model to fit correlated data. In this chapter, we use an approach other than using a common factor and incorporate a series of weights or design effects to account for the correlation.

5.2 Definition and Notation

To make the information in this chapter clearer and simpler, it is worth looking at Gene Shackman's discussion on *design effects* which he presented at Albany Chapter of American Statistical Association, March 24, 2001. Below is the text of his exposito:

J. R. Wilson et al., *Modeling Binary Correlated Responses*, ICSA Book Series in Statistics, https://doi.org/10.1007/978-3-031-62427-8_5

Cluster sampling is commonly used, rather than simple random sampling, mainly as a means of saving money, for example, the population is spread out, and the researcher cannot sample from everywhere. However, "respondents in the same cluster are likely to be somewhat similar to one another." As a result, in a clustered sample, "Selecting an additional member from the same cluster adds less new information than would a completely independent selection." Thus, for example, in single stage cluster samples, the sample is not as varied as it would be in a random sample, so that the effective sample size is reduced. The loss of effectiveness by the use of cluster sampling, instead of simple random sampling, is the *design effect*.

The design effect is basically the ratio of the actual variance, under the sampling method actually used, to the variance computed under the assumption of simple random sampling. For an example, "The interpretation of a value of (design effect) of, say, 3.0, is that the sample variance is 3 times bigger than it would be if the survey were based on the same sample size but selected randomly. An alternative interpretation is that only one-third as many sample cases would be needed to measure the given statistic if a simple random sample were used instead of the cluster sample with its (design effect) of 3.0." The main components of the design effect are the intraclass correlation and the cluster sample sizes. Thus, the design effect is $DEFF = 1 + \delta(n - 1)$, where DEFF is the design effect, δ is the intraclass correlation for the statistic in question, and n is the average size of the cluster. Therefore, the design effect increases as the cluster sizes increase and as the intraclass correlation increases. The intraclass correlation represents the likelihood that two elements in the same cluster have the same value, for a given statistic, relative to two elements chosen completely at random in the population. A value of 0.05 is interpreted, therefore, to mean that the elements in the cluster are about 5% more likely to have the same value than if the two elements were chosen at random in the survey. The smaller the value, the better the overall reliability of the sample estimate will be.

Design effects vary from survey to survey and, even within the same survey, will vary from question to question. For example, "respondents who live near each other (in the same sampled cluster) are likely to have similar poverty characteristics but are not likely to have similar disability characteristics." Similarly, if the sampling unit is households, the design effect would be high for characteristics that are the same for all members of the household (e.g., ethnicity) and would be low for characteristics that are different for different members of the household (e.g., education, age).

Researchers also use the DEFT, which is the square root of the DEFF. The DEFT may be used to reduce variability, since the DEFT is less variable than the DEFF. The DEFT can also be used directly to estimate confidence intervals.

The DEFT (square root of DEFF) shows how much the sample standard error, and consequently the confidence intervals, increases. Thus, for example, if the DEFT is 3, the confidence intervals have to be three times as large as they would for a simple random sample. In sum, using a cluster sample generally requires either a larger sample size than a SRS or using a wider confidence interval. The design effect is used to determine how much larger the sample size or confidence interval needs to be. The second handout lists a number of studies, and some information about the studies, including the sampling design (if the information is available), the design effects, and intraclass correlations found in these studies. The handout also lists some reports that describe information about design effects. In general, for a well-designed study, the design effect usually ranges from 1 to 3. It is not uncommon, however, for the design effect to be much larger, up to 7 or 8, or even up to 30.

5.3 Exploratory Analyses

Researchers often use sample survey methodology to obtain samples from local populations and to estimate parameters intended to be representative of the overall population. We fit logistic regression models based on the covariates measured in the survey data. For example, the National Health and Nutrition Examination Survey (NHANES) is a program of studies designed to assess the health and nutritional status of adults and children in the United States. "The survey is unique in that it combines interviews and physical examinations. It is the National Center for Health Statistics (NCHS) most in-depth and logistically complex survey, operating out of mobile examination centers that travel to randomly selected sites throughout the country to assess the health and nutritional status of Americans. This survey combines personal interviews with standardized physical examinations, diagnostic procedures, and laboratory tests to obtain information about diagnosed and undiagnosed conditions; growth and development, including overweight and obesity; diet and nutrition; risk factors; and environmental exposures" (http://www.cdc.gov/nchs/nhanes.htm). We looked at the following example:

5.3.1 Treatment for Osteoporosis

This example uses the *demoadv* dataset, a subset from National Health and Nutrition Examination Survey (NHANES) database (Centers for Disease Control, 2009). We desired the association between calcium supplement use (*anycalsup-1 use any supplement*) and the likelihood of receiving treatment for osteoporosis (*treatosteo*) among participants, aged 20 years old and older after controlling for selected covariates. The covariates include gender (*riagendr—1 for men and 2 for women*), age (*ridageyr—age at screening*), race/ethnicity (*ridreth1*), and body mass index (*bmxbmi*). Information on use of vitamin, mineral, herbal, and other dietary supplements originate from all the NHANES participants during the household interview.

Stage 1: Primary sampling units (PSUs) are selected from strata defined by geography and proportions of minority populations. These are mostly single counties or, in a few cases, groups of contiguous counties selected with probability proportional to a measure of size (PPS). Most strata contain two PSUs. Additional stages of sampling are performed to select various types of secondary sampling units (SSUs), namely, the segments, households, and individuals that are selected in Stages 2, 3, and 4.

Stage 2: The PSUs are divided into segments (generally city blocks or their equivalent). As with each PSU, sample segments are selected with PPS.

Stage 3: Households within each segment were listed, and a sample is randomly drawn. In geographic areas where the proportion of age, ethnic, or income groups selected for over-sampling is high, the probability of selection for those groups is greater than in other areas.

Stage 4: Individuals are chosen to participate in NHANES from a list of all persons residing in selected households. Individuals are drawn at random within designated age-sex-race/ethnicity screening sub-domains. Between one and two persons on average are selected from a household. A schematic diagram is as follows (Fig. 5.1).

SAS User's Group International (SUGI) 27 provides information suitable for logistic regression on survey data. Survey data researchers, among others, have addressed the problems by using a standard logistic regression in sample surveys (Rao & Scott, 1981; Scott & Rao, 1981; William, 1982). Others include Binder (1981, 1983), Roberts et al. (1987), Skinner et al. (1989), Morel (1989), Wilson (1989), and Lehtonen and Pahkinen (1995).

SUGI 27 suggests that due to the variability of characteristics among items in the population, researchers apply scientific sample designs in the sample selection process to reduce the risk of a distorted view of the population. They will make inferences about the population based on the information from the sample survey data. Rao and Scott (1981) laid the foundation for understanding that, in order to make

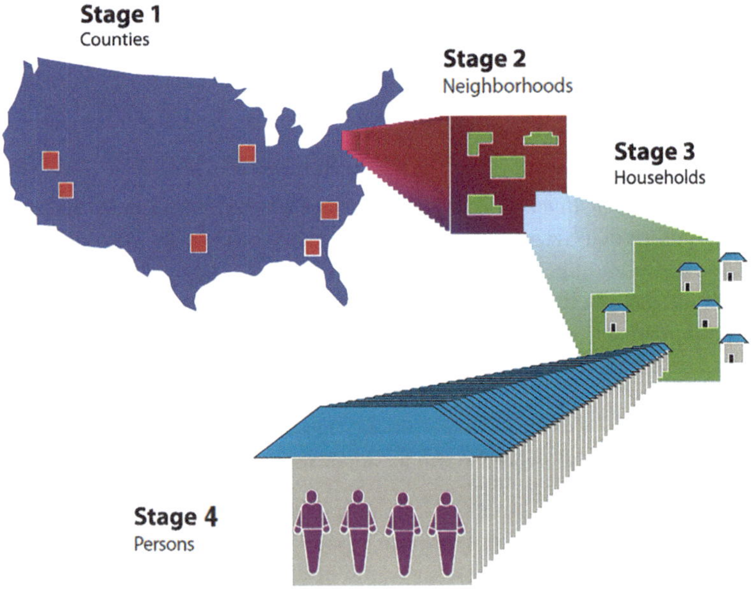

Fig. 5.1 NHANES sampling procedure. (Image source: https://www.cdc.gov/nchs/nhanes/participant/participant-selected.htm)

statistically valid inferences for the population, researchers must incorporate the sample design in the data analysis. We looked at procedures that allowed us to fit logistic regression models to survey data. We needed it to fit linear logistic regression models for binary response survey data by the method of maximum likelihood. For our analysis, we incorporated complex survey sample designs, including designs with stratification, clustering, and unequal weighting.

5.4 Statistical Model

Complex surveys usually comprise data that originated based on sample designs that have adjusted for nonresponse and differing probabilities of selection. Complex samples differ from simple random samples (SRS) in that SRS designs assume independence of observations while complex samples do not. Statistics produced by the default in most cases with programs and procedures assume a simple random sample and result in underestimation of variances when analyzing data that arise from complex samples. In such situations, we are more likely to conclude there is significance when in fact there is not. Therefore, the analysis of data from complex surveys should include specific calculation of variance estimates that account for these sample characteristics (National Center for Health Statistics, 2005). Also, weights are used to adjust for the nonresponse and for differing probabilities of selection used in analyses. We used survey procedures incorporating weights, strata, and cluster variables as they ensured that we had variance estimates that incorporate the complex sample design and reflect the inflation of the estimate due to the design effect.

In Chap. 3, we use methods to compute statistics under the assumption that a sample is drawn from an infinite population through simple random sampling. However, most sample survey data are collected from a finite population with a probability-based complex sample design (Rao & Scott, 1981). Logistic regression modeling is often used to profile certain respondents based on the binary outcome with input variables for survey data. However, there are many examples of logistic regression in surveys that can be found (Korn & Graubard, 1999). The link function (logit) in logistic regression combines the probabilities of an outcome with a function of a linear combination of the explanatory variables. As it is customary in the analysis of survey data to make statistically valid inferences for the population, the sample design used to obtain the sample data is incorporated in the data analysis. The use of complex sampling schemes to obtain the data impacts the standard error of the estimates.

When a complex sample design is used to draw a sample from a finite population, the sample design is incorporated in the analysis of the survey data in order to make statistically valid inferences for the finite population. This results in a weighted logistic regression model for binary observations. The weighted logistic regression model accommodates three common types of complex survey data, as listed and explained below.

1. Survey weights: Survey data are often published along with weights for each observation. For example, if a survey intentionally over-samples a particular type of case, weights can be used to correct for the overrepresentation of that type of case in the dataset. Survey weights come in two forms:
   (a) Probability weights report the probability that each case is drawn from the population. For each stratum or cluster, this is computed as the number of observations in the sample drawn from that group divided by the number of observations in the population in the group.
   (b) Sampling weights are the inverse of the probability weights.
2. Strata/cluster identification: A complex survey dataset may include variables that identify the strata or cluster from which observations are drawn. For stratified random sampling designs, observations may be nested in different strata. There are two ways to employ these identifiers:
   (a) Use finite population corrections to specify the total number of cases in the stratum or cluster from which each observation was drawn.
   (b) For stratified random sampling designs, use the raw strata IDs to compute sampling weights from the data.
3. Replication weights: To preserve the anonymity of survey participants, some surveys exclude strata and cluster IDs from the public data and instead release only precomputed replicate weights.

5.5 Analysis of Data

In this section, we use the data from NHANES to demonstrate the fit of weighted logistic regression models. Our binary response variable of interest is receiving treatment for osteoporosis (*treatosteo*). We want to know how calcium supplement use (*anycalsup*) impacts the probability of receiving treatment for osteoporosis (*treatosteo*) among participants, aged 20 years old and older, after controlling for gender (*riagendr*), age (*ridageyr*), race/ethnicity *(ridreth1*), and body mass index (*bmxbmi*). The variables are coded as

AGEGRP (1 = '20–39' 2 = '40–59' 3 = '> = 60';) and YESNO (1 = 'Yes' 2 = 'No') and 1 = 'Used any calcium supp' 2 = 'No supp use'; with GENDER 1 = 'Male' 2 = 'Female'. Information on use of vitamin, mineral, herbal, and other dietary supplements was collected from all NHANES participants during the household interview. We present two models:

1. Weighted logistic regression model, demonstrating the assignment of weights without giving heed to strata or clusters.
2. Weighted logistic regression model, incorporating weights while identifying the strata or clusters and adjusting the weights accordingly.

5.5.1 *Weighted Logistic Regression Model with Survey Weights*

A weighted logistic regression model was fitted. These required weights are contained in a weight variable referred to as *newweight*. This allows the units to have different levels of importance in the model fitting.

5.5.2 *Weighted Logistic Regression Model with Survey Weights Using SAS Program*

We fit a weighted logistic regression model using SAS. Both PROC LOGISTIC and PROC SURVEYLOGISTIC were used. While they use the same method to compute the maximum likelihood estimates of the regression coefficients, the standard errors are different and the methods used to compute them differ. The logistic regression model with survey data incorporates the variance as applicable for stratification, clustering, and unequal weighting. The PROC SURVEYLOGISTIC uses the results of variances within each stratum and then pools the variance estimates together to give a joint estimate. An adjustment can also be obtained in the variance estimation to reduce the bias when the sample size is small and the sample is drawn without replacement (Morel, 1989).

Model 1: Weighted Logistic Regression Model

```
proc logistic data=work.chap5;
weight newweight;
class age riagendr anycalsup bmigrp/param=ref;
model treatosteo =anycalsup riagendr age bmigrp;
run;
```

Comment This runs the weighted logistic regression model. The weights are contained in the variable *newweight*. Param = ref. refers to the categorical variables and their reference category.

SAS Output

The logistic procedure	
Model information	
Dataset	WORK.CHAPTER5
Response variable	treatOSTEO
Number of response levels	2
Weight variable	Newweight
Model	Binary logit
Optimization technique	Fisher's scoring
Number of observations read	5023

The logistic procedure	
Number of observations used	4623
Sum of weights read	2.049E8
Sum of weights used	2.0111E8

Comment Not all the observations are used. Most likely not all variables have complete information.

Response profile			
Ordered value	treatOSTEO	Total frequency	Total weight
1	0	4385	192516945
2	1	238	8597732
Probability modeled is treatOSTEO = '0'.			

Comment We are modeling the probability that they are not receiving treatment for osteoporosis. As we will see, it is very easy to model receiving treatment for osteoporosis by changing the signs in the logistic regression model. There are 4485 cases of 0 and 238 of 1.

Class level information			
Class	Value	Design variables	
age	1	1	0
	2	0	1
	3	0	0
RIAGENDR	1	1	
	2	0	
ANYCALSUP	1	1	
	2	0	
bmigrp	1	1	0
	2	0	1
	3	0	0

Comment Since these are class (categorical) variables, we need to present them as a series of binary variables (see Sect. 1.6). So we have (Age = 3 − 1) + (Riagendr = 2 − 1) + (Anycalsup = 2 − 1) + (bmigrp = 3 − 1) = 6 + intercept parameter = 7.

Model convergence status		
Convergence criterion (GCONV = 1E-8) satisfied		
Model fit statistics		
Criterion	Intercept only	Intercept and covariates
AIC	71029139	52689533
SC	71029145	52689578
−2 Log L	71029137	52689519

Testing global null hypothesis: Beta = 0			
Test	Chi-square	DF	Pr > ChiSq
Likelihood ratio	18339617.9	6	<0.0001
Score	18408564.5	6	<0.0001
Wald	10461411.8	6	<0.0001

Comment The covariates collectively have a significant impact on nontreatment of osteoporosis. The model fit statistics provide values with the covariates and without the covariates.

Type 3 analysis of effects			
Effect	DF	Wald chi-square	Pr > ChiSq
ANYCALSUP	1	342591.094	<0.0001
RIAGENDR	1	3319345.29	<0.0001
age	2	6413787.54	<0.0001
bmigrp	2	202151.263	<0.0001

Analysis of maximum likelihood estimates						
Parameter		DF	Estimate	Standard error	Wald chi-square	Pr > ChiSq
Intercept		1	1.7340	0.000939	3410931.30	<0.0001
ANYCALSUP	1	1	−0.4820	0.000823	342591.094	<0.0001
RIAGENDR	1	1	2.1072	0.00116	3319345.29	<0.0001
age	1	1	4.0852	0.00229	3174953.84	<0.0001
age	2	1	1.6604	0.000834	3965962.69	<0.0001
bmigrp	1	1	−0.3657	0.000925	156354.817	<0.0001
bmigrp	2	1	−0.0323	0.000945	1166.7900	<0.0001

Comment The fitted logistic regression model is

$$\text{logit}\, P_{no\,treat}) = 1.734 - 0.482 Anycalsup\,(= use\,calcium) + 2.107 Riagendr\,(= male)$$
$$+ 4.085 Age_1 + 1.660 Age_2 - 0.366 bmigrp_1 - 0.032 bmigrp_2$$

All the covariates are significant in the model. Those who used calcium supplement (ANYCALSUP = 1) are more likely to have treatOSTEO = '1'.

Odds ratio estimates			
Effect	Point estimate	95% Wald confidence limits	
ANYCALSUP 1 vs 2	0.618	0.617	0.619
RIAGENDR 1 vs 2	8.225	8.206	8.244
age 1 vs 3	59.455	59.188	59.723
age 2 vs 3	5.262	5.253	5.270
bmigrp 1 vs 3	0.694	0.692	0.695
bmigrp 2 vs 3	0.968	0.966	0.970

Comment The odds ratios are all significant. For example, age 2 vs 3 with odds 5.270 says that those in age class =2 are 5.27 times more likely not to have the treatment than those in age class = 3.

Association of predicted probabilities and observed responses			
Percent concordant	85.4	Somers' D	0.745
Percent discordant	11.0	Gamma	0.772
Percent tied	3.6	Tau-a	0.073
Pairs	1043630	c	0.872

5.5.3 Weighted Logistic Regression Model with Survey Weights Using SPSS Program

SPSS Program

Model 1: Weighted logistic regression model
The SPSS Syntax for weighted logistic regression cannot be done with the pull-down menus because there is no weight option in *Binary Logistic* in SPSS. First fit with no weights. *To run a set of code in SPSS for weighted logistic regression, follow these steps:

```
Step 1:
Click "File" on the toolbar
Select "New"
Click "Syntax"

Step 2:
Paste the following code into the new Syntax window:
WEIGHT BY newweight.
LOGISTIC REGRESSION VARIABLES treatOSTEO
/METHOD=ENTER ANYCALSUP RIAGENDR age bmigrp
/CONTRAST (age)=Indicator
/CONTRAST (bmigrp)=Indicator
/CONTRAST (RIAGENDR)=Indicator
/CONTRAST (ANYCALSUP)=Indicator
/CRITERIA=PIN(.05) POUT(.10) ITERATE(20) CUT(.5).

Step 3:
Click "Run" on the toolbar
Click "All"
```

SPSS Output

Case processing summary

Unweighted cases[a]		N	Percent
Selected cases	Included in analysis	4623	45.7
	Missing cases	5499	54.3
	Total	10122	100.0
Unselected cases		0	0.0
Total		10122	100.0

[a]If weight is in effect, see classification table for the total number of cases

Comment There were 5499 missing cases that are excluded.

Dependent variable encoding

Original value	Internal value
0	0
1	1

Comment The coding is helpful in determining the numerator and the denominator in the equation.

Categorical variables codings				
		Frequency	Parameter coding	
			(1)	(2)
bmigrp	1	1465	1.000	0.000
	2	1624	0.000	1.000
	3	1534	0.000	0.000
age	1	1626	1.000	0.000
	2	1306	0.000	1.000
	3	1691	0.000	0.000
RIAGENDR	1	2228	1.000	
	2	2395	0.000	
ANYCALSUP	1	2155	1.000	
	2	2468	0.000	

Comment The distribution of observations in each category of each covariate is given. For example, there are 2228 men and 2395 women with complete data to be included in this model. There are 3 × 3 × 2 × 2 = 36 subpopulations. However, the missing data made many of the combinations useless.

Block 1: method = enter.

Omnibus tests of model coefficients				
		Chi-square	DF	Sig.
Step 1	Step	479.352	6	0.000
	Block	479.352	6	0.000
	Model	479.352	6	0.000

Comment SPSS with the "Enter" option provides information as it reaches the solution.

Model summary			
Step	−2 Log likelihood	Cox and Snell R-square	Nagelkerke R-square
1	1396.247[a]	0.098	0.295

[a]Estimation terminated at iteration number 9 because parameter estimates changed by less than 0.001

Comment These model summary statistics talk about the fit of the model. There are varying views over the use of these statistics.

Variables in the equation							
		B	S.E.	Wald	DF	Sig.	Exp(B)
Step 1[a]	ANYCALSUP(1)	0.789	0.158	24.906	1	0.000	2.200
	RIAGENDR(1)	−2.008	0.202	98.849	1	0.000	0.134
	age			104.071	2	0.000	
	age(1)	−4.752	0.713	44.426	1	0.000	0.009
	age(2)	−1.519	0.189	64.594	1	0.000	0.219
	bmigrp			7.218	2	0.027	
	bmigrp(1)	0.470	0.179	6.882	1	0.009	1.601
	bmigrp(2)	0.170	0.179	0.910	1	0.340	1.186
	Constant	−2.118	0.176	143.992	1	0.000	0.120

Comment The fitted logistic regression model logit(P_{treat})=−2.118+0.789Anycalsup−2.008*Riagendr* −4.752Age_1 −1.519Age_2 + 0.470$bmigrp_1$ + 0.170$bmigrp_2$. These variables are significant in the model.

Variables in the equation			
		95% C.I. for EXP(B)	
		Lower	Upper
Step 1[a]	ANYCALSUP(1)	1.614	2.999
	RIAGENDR(1)	0.090	0.199
	age		
	age(1)	0.002	0.035
	age(2)	0.151	0.317
	bmigrp		
	bmigrp(1)	1.126	2.275
	bmigrp(2)	0.835	1.683
	Constant		

[a]Variable(s) entered on step 1: ANYCALSUP, RIAGENDR, age, bmigrp

Comment The values for the logit estimates have different signs due to modeling the event = 1. This changes the interpretation of the odds ratios in association to the change in likelihood of an event based upon a different reference category.

Comment Note the weight variable defined before the analysis syntax. These weights are user defined and available from, in this example, the NHANES website. The SPSS Syntax for weighted logistic regression cannot be done with the pull-down menus because there is no weight option in binary logistic in SPSS.

*To run a set of code in SPSS, follow these steps:

```
Step 1:
Click "File" on the toolbar
Select "New"
Click "Syntax"

Step 2:
Paste the code into the new Syntax window

Step 3:
Click "Run" on the toolbar
Click "All"
```

Logistic Regression

Case processing summary

Unweighted cases[a]		N	Percent
Selected cases	Included in analysis	4623	97.8
	Missing cases	104	2.2
	Total	4727	100.0
Unselected cases		0	0.0
Total		4727	100.0

[a]If weight is in effect, see classification table for the total number of cases

Dependent variable encoding

Original value	Internal value
0	0
1	1

Classification table[a]

	Observed		Predicted		
			treatOSTEO		Percentage correct
			0	1	
Step 1	treatOSTEO	0	192516945	0	100.0
		1	8597732	0	0.0
	Overall percentage				95.7

[a]The cut value is 0.500

Variables in the equation							
		B	S.E.	Wald	DF	Sig.	Exp(B)
Step 1[a]	ANYCALSUP(1)	0.482	0.001	342590.806	1	0.000	1.619
	RIAGENDR(1)	−2.107	0.001	3319343.261	1	0.000	0.122
	age			6413762.099	2	0.000	
	age(1)	−4.085	0.002	3174916.020	1	0.000	0.017
	age(2)	−1.660	0.001	3965962.639	1	0.000	0.190
	bmigrp			202151.111	2	0.000	
	bmigrp(1)	0.366	0.001	156354.703	1	0.000	1.442
	bmigrp(2)	0.032	0.001	1166.789	1	0.000	1.033
	Constant	−1.734	0.001	3410929.320	1	0.000	0.177

[a]Variable(s) entered on step 1: ANYCALSUP, RIAGENDR, age, bmigrp

Comment The fitted logistic regression model is

$$Logit\left(P_{no\,treat}\right) = 1.734 - 0.482 Anycalsup + 2.107 Riagendr + 4.085 Age_1 + 1.660 Age_2$$
$$- 0.366 bmigrp_1 - 0.032 bmigrp_2$$

5.5.4 *Weighted Logistic Regression Model with Survey Weights Using R Program*

R Program

```
> data1$ANYCALSUP.f <- factor(data1$ANYCALSUP)
> data1$RIAGENDR.f <- factor(data1$RIAGENDR)
> data1$age.f <- factor(data1$age)
> data1$bmigrp.f <- factor(data1$bmigrp)
> glm.out=glm(treatOSTEO ~ ANYCALSUP.f + RIAGENDR.f + age.f +
bmigrp.f, family=binomial(logit), data=data1)
> summary(glm.out)
Call:
glm(formula = treatOSTEO ~ ANYCALSUP.f + RIAGENDR.f + age.f +
bmigrp.f, family = binomial(logit), data = data1)
```

Comment We fit the unweighted logistic regression model.

R Output

```
DEVIANCE RESIDUALS:
  Min        1Q      Median     3Q        Max
-0.8405  -0.2873  -0.1245  -0.0456   3.4882
COEFFICIENTS:
                 ESTIMATE   STD. ERROR   Z VALUE    PR(>|z|)
(Intercept)     -7.6188    0.7377      -10.328   < 2e-16 ***
ANYCALSUP.f1    -0.7885    0.1580      -4.991    6.02e-07 ***
RIAGENDR.f1      2.007     0.2019       9.942    < 2e-16 ***
age.f1           3.2327    0.7286       4.437    9.14e-06 ***
age.f2           4.7520    0.7129       6.666    2.64e-11 ***
bmigrp.f1       -0.3000    0.1701      -1.763    0.07784 .
bmigrp.f2       -0.4704    0.1793      -2.623    0.00871 **
---
Signif. codes:  0 '***' 0.001 '**' 0.01 '*' 0.05 '.' 0.1 ' ' 1
(Dispersion parameter for binomial family taken to be 1)
Null deviance: 1875.6 on 4622 degrees of freedom
Residual deviance: 1396.2 on 4616 degrees of freedom
(400 observations deleted due to missingness)
AIC: 1410.2
Number of Fisher Scoring iterations: 9
```

Comment The fitted unweighted logistic regression model is

$$Logit\left(P_{no\,treat}\right) = -7.619 - 0.789 Anycalsup + 2.008 Riagendr + 3.233 Age_1 + 4.752 Age_2 - 0.300 bmigrp_1 - 0.470 bmigrp_2.$$

```
> design1<-svydesign(ids=~0, weights=data1$newweight, data=data1)
> svyglm.out=svyglm(treatOSTEO ~ ANYCALSUP.f + RIAGENDR.f + age.f
+ bmigrp.f, family=quasibinomial(logit), data=data1,
design=design1)
> summary(svyglm.out)
Call:
svyglm(formula = treatOSTEO ~ ANYCALSUP.f + RIAGENDR.f + age.f +
    bmigrp.f, family = quasibinomial(logit), data = data1, design
= design1)
Survey design:
svydesign(ids = ~0, weights = data1$newweight, data = data1)
```

Comment We fit the weighted logistic regression model.

```
Coefficients:
                  Estimate     Std. Error   t value   Pr(>|t|)
(Intercept)       -7.0787      0.7504       -9.433    < 2e-16 ***
ANYCALSUP.f1      -0.4820      0.1954       -2.467    0.0137 *
RIAGENDR.f1       2.1072       0.2265        9.301    < 2e-16 ***
age.f1            2.4248       0.7423        3.267    0.0011 **
age.f2            4.0852       0.7230        5.651    1.69e-08 ***
bmigrp.f1        -0.3334       0.1964       -1.698    0.0896 .
bmigrp.f2        -0.3657       0.2271       -1.611    0.1073

---Signif. codes:  0 '***' 0.001 '**' 0.01 '*' 0.05 '.' 0.1 ' ' 1
(Dispersion parameter for quasibinomial family taken to be 0.9146361)
Number of Fisher Scoring iterations: 8.
```

Comment The fitted weighted logistic regression is

$$Logit\left(P_{no\,treat}\right) = -7.619 - 0.789 Anycalsup + 2.008 Riagendr + 3.233 Age_1 + 4.752 Age_2 - 0.300 bmigrp_1 - 0.470 bmigrp_2$$

The BMI is not significant in the model.

5.5.5 Weighted Logistic Regression Model with Strata and Clusters Identified

We fit the weighted logistic regression model while we include the identity of the strata and the clusters through their weights. We use PROC Surveylogistic to fit these data.

SAS Program

```
proc surveylogistic data=work.chap5;
stratum sdmvstra;
cluster sdmvpsu;
weight newweight;
class age riagendr anycalsup bmigrp /param=ref;
model treatosteo =anycalsup riagendr age bmigrp;
run;
quit;
```

Comment The results are similar to the earlier logistic regression model fit with survey weights. However, the covariate body mass index showed no significant contribution, and the covariate calcium use was not as significant. The stratum is identified through sdmvstra and cluster is identified through sdmvpsu.

SAS Output

The SURVEYLOGISTIC procedure	
Model information	
Dataset	WORK.CHAPTER6
Response variable	treatOSTEO
Number of response levels	2
Stratum variable	SDMVSTRA
Number of strata	15
Cluster variable	SDMVPSU
Number of clusters	30
Weight variable	Newweight
Model	Binary logit
Optimization technique	Fisher's scoring
Variance adjustment	Degrees of freedom (DF)

Variance estimation	
Method	Taylor series
Variance adjustment	Degrees of freedom (DF)
Number of observations read	5023
Number of observations used	4623
Sum of weights read	2.049E8
Sum of weights used	2.0111E8

Comment The variance estimation which is a key component for analysis was done based on the Taylor series method. The sum of the weights used is seen below: $2.0111 \times 10^8 = 192516945 + 8597732$. These are the same weights in Model 1.

Response profile			
Ordered value	treatOSTEO	Total frequency	Total weight
1	0	4385	192516945
2	1	238	8597732
Probability modeled is treatOSTEO = '0'.			

Comment The model converged.

Model fit statistics		
Criterion	Intercept only	Intercept and covariates
AIC	71029139	52689533
SC	71029145	52689578
−2 Log L	71029137	52689519

Testing global null hypothesis: Beta = 0			
Test	Chi-square	DF	Pr > ChiSq
Likelihood ratio	18339617.9	6	<0.0001
Score	18408564.5	6	<0.0001
Wald	1201.6698	6	<0.0001

Comment The results in this Model 2 have a simultaneous significant impact on no treatment as in Model 1.

Type 3 analysis of effects			
Effect	DF	Wald chi-square	Pr > ChiSq
ANYCALSUP	1	5.5436	0.0185
RIAGENDR	1	138.1695	<0.0001
age	2	697.7815	<0.0001
bmigrp	2	3.3351	0.1887

Comment While these covariates (Anycalsup, Riagendr, Age, and Bmigrp) are significant, the additional effect of BMIGRP is not significant.

Analysis of maximum likelihood estimates						
Parameter		DF	Estimate	Standard error	Wald chi-square	Pr > ChiSq
Intercept		1	1.7340	0.2019	73.7907	<0.0001
ANYCALSUP	1	1	−0.4820	0.2047	5.5436	0.0185
RIAGENDR	1	1	2.1072	0.1793	138.1695	<0.0001
age	1	1	4.0852	0.1917	454.1055	<0.0001
age	2	1	1.6604	0.2245	54.6801	<0.0001
bmigrp	1	1	−0.3657	0.2007	3.3207	0.0684
bmigrp	2	1	−0.0323	0.1832	0.0310	0.8602

Odds ratio estimates			
Effect	Point estimate	95% Wald confidence limits	
ANYCALSUP 1 vs 2	0.618	0.413	0.922
RIAGENDR 1 vs 2	8.225	5.788	11.688
age 1 vs 3	59.455	40.833	86.570
age 2 vs 3	5.262	3.388	8.171
bmigrp 1 vs 3	0.694	0.468	1.028
bmigrp 2 vs 3	0.968	0.676	1.386

Comment Correspondingly the odds ratios are significant in all cases except with BMIGRP.

Association of predicted probabilities and observed responses			
Percent concordant	85.4	Somers' D	0.745
Percent discordant	11.0	Gamma	0.772
Percent tied	3.6	Tau-a	0.073
Pairs	1043630	c	0.872

Comment The BMI_Grp is not significant in the model. The fitted weighted logistic regression model is as follows:

$$\begin{aligned}\text{Logit}\left(P_{no\,treat}\right) = 1.734 - 0.482 Anycalsup + 2.107 Riagendr + 4.085 Age_1 \\ + 1.660 Age_2 - 0.366 bmigrp_1 - 0.032 bmigrp_2.\end{aligned}$$

5.5.6 *Comparison of Weighted Logistic Regression Models*

We fitted a weighted logistic regression model with the set of weights (Model#1) and another with weights based on the strata and clusters (Model#2) to which the observations belong. The parameter estimates are the same in both models, but the variances are different. The ratio of the standard errors is given in Table 5.1.

Model #2 took into account the strata and the clusters, so it is expected that the variance will be greater.

5.6 Conclusion

When binary data are obtained from clusters of different sizes, there are some methods more efficient to use other than a common dispersion factor as seen in Chap. 4. So instead of forcing a common factor on the data, one can use the weighted logistic regression model. It is possible to fit the varying clusters as a categorical variable in the model. If the clusters are the only ones of interest, then one may need to include dummy variables to address the clusters. When you have survey data, the estimates

Table 5.1 Standard error estimates and ratio of standard errors

	Model_1	Model_2	Ratio = Model_2/Model_1
Intercept	0.000939	0.2019	215.0159744
Anycalsup	0.000823	0.2047	248.7241798
Riagendr	0.00116	0.1793	154.5689655
Age_1	0.00229	0.1917	83.71179039
Age_2	0.000834	0.2245	269.1846523
Bmi_grp	0.000925	0.2007	216.972973
Bmi_grp	0.000945	0.1832	193.8624339

are affected as opposed to if you had assumed the observations were independent. Ignoring the correlation present results in the variance being underestimated; thus, estimates may be presented as significant when in fact they are not.

5.7 Related Examples

The initial year of the High School and Beyond data survey was conducted in the. spring of 1980. The survey design included a highly stratified national probability sample of 1106 secondary schools as the first-stage units of selection. In the second stage, 36 seniors and 36 sophomores were selected per school. Sampling rates for each stratum were set so as to select in each stratum the number of schools needed to satisfy study design criteria regarding minimum sample sizes for certain types of schools. As a result, some schools had a very high probability of inclusion. The total number of schools selected for the sample was 1122, from a frame of 24,725 schools with grades 10, 12, or both. The data concentrated on the TV viewing habits of black and white seniors in alternative and regular Catholic schools in the west north central region. One can fit a weighted logistic regression model to model those who watch lots of television vs. those who do not.

Wilson, J. R., & Wilson, P. M. (1991). A comparison of chi-squared statistics for testing homogeneity of survey data: High school and beyond survey. *Journal of Applied Statistics*, *18*(2), 203–213.

References

Binder, D. A. (1981). On the variances of asymptotically normal estimators from complex surveys. *Survey Methodology, 7*, 157–170.

Binder, D. A. (1983). On the variances of asymptotically normal estimators from complex surveys. *International Statistical Review, 51*, 279–292.

Center for Disease Control and Prevention. (2009). *National health and nutrition examination survey*. Atlanta GA US Department of Health and Human Services, Senters of Disease Control.

Korn, E., & Graubard, B. (1999). *Analysis of health survey*. Wiley.

Lehtonen, R., & Pahkinen, E. (1995). *Practical methods for design and analysis of complex surveys*. Wiley.

Morel, G. (1989). Logistic regression under complex survey designs. *Survey Methodology, 15*, 203–223.

National Center for Health Statistics. (2005). *Analytic and reporting guidelines:* The National Health and Nutrition Examination Survey (NHANES) Centers for Disease Control and Prevention Hyattsville, MD.

Rao, J. N. K., & Scott, A. J. (1981). The analysis of categorical data from complex surveys. *Journal of the American Statistical Association, 76*, 221–230.

Rao, J. N. K., & Scott, A. J. (1984). On Chi-Square tests for multiway contingency tables with cell proportions estimated from survey data. *Annals of Statistics, 12*, 46–60.

Roberts, G., Rao, J. N. K., & Kumar, S. (1987). Logistic regression analysis of sample survey data. *Biometrika, 74*, 1–12.

Scott, A. J., & Rao, J. N. K. (1981). Chi-squared tests for contingency tables with proportions estimated from survey data. In D. Krewski, R. Platek, & J. N. K. Rao (Eds.), *Current topics in survey sampling* (pp. 247–266). Academic.

Skinner, C. J., Holt, D., & Smith, T. M. F. (1989). *Analysis of complex surveys*. Wiley.

Williams, D. A. (1982). Extra-binomial variation in logistic linear models. *Applied Statistics, 31*(783), 144–148.

Wilson, J. R. (1989). Chi-square tests for overdispersion with multiparameter estimates. *Journal of Royal Statistics Society Series C, Applied Statistics, 38*(3), 441–454.

Chapter 6
Generalized Estimating Equations Logistic Regression

6.1 Motivating Example

6.1.1 Description of the Rehospitalization Issues

Longitudinal datasets usually consist of repeated measurements on a response variable, often accompanied by a set of covariates for each of the subjects/units. However, longitudinal datasets are problematic because they inherently show correlation due to a subject's repeated set of measurements. For example, one might expect that a correlation exists between a patient's health status and its progress over time, or a student's grade performance and its progress over time, but it does not allow us to draw a correlative relationship between the two. In looking at the longitudinal datasets, consider this example regarding hospitalization, an important issue for health insurance reimbursement. A hospital has obtained information about rehospitalization for 1625 patients on 3 successive occasions. The CFO of the hospital wants to know if there are some indicators to help determine the probability of rehospitalization within 30 days. The data are given in the *Medicare* dataset (https://www.public.asu.edu/~jeffreyw). The covariates under consideration are total number of diagnoses, total number of procedures, length of previous stay, and whether or not they had coronary atherosclerosis.

Study Hypotheses
The CFO is particularly interested in total number of diagnoses at hospitalization (NDX), total number of procedures performed previously (NPR), length of stay at the previous stay (LOS), and whether or not they had coronary atherosclerosis (DX101) as they impact rehospitalization. By analyzing the data, the CFO wants to know the probability of a patient being rehospitalized within 30 days of release, based on the number of prescriptions, the total number of procedures he/she has had, the length of his/her previous stay, and whether or not he/she has coronary atherosclerosis.

J. R. Wilson et al., *Modeling Binary Correlated Responses*, ICSA Book Series in Statistics, https://doi.org/10.1007/978-3-031-62427-8_6

6.2 Definition and Notation

Longitudinal studies are studies in which the outcome variable is repeatedly measured on two or more occasions over time.

Clustered data are data created with a common mechanism. The units are not independently and identically distributed but rather come in groups or clusters that consist of units which are correlated. Such units of data are put into any number of distinct groups or "clusters" within a particular study (Galbraith et al., 2010). Additionally, the sampling units in a study are grouped into clusters if they share a common feature.

Repeated measures data consist of data which are longitudinal or clustered. Most researchers refer to repeated measures data to denote those data that are taken repeatedly over time, as well as those not taken over time, but have otherwise correlated outcome data; we will do likewise. Thus, we use the term "repeated measures" to include both longitudinal and clustered data.

A *marginal model*, also known as a population-averaged model, is used when the researcher is modeling the mean of the distribution of the population of responses and wishes to do so as a function of the covariates. From these models, researchers make conclusions about comparisons between subpopulations that differ according to chosen covariates.

Generalized estimating equations (GEE) is a method used for obtaining estimates of the coefficient when analyzing correlated observations without relying on a joint distribution of the responses which is usually unknown. The method is usually used for cases which could normally be modeled as generalized linear models (GLMs), but because of correlation among the observations, it cannot (http://support.sas.com/rnd/app/da/new/dagee.html) (Hardin & Hilbe, 2003; Liang & Zeger, 1986).

A *consistent estimator* is one which, if allowed to be computed each time with a larger sample size, will result in the value it was set to estimate. More so, a sequence of estimators for a parameter is said to be consistent (or asymptotically consistent) if this sequence converges in probability to the parameter. It means that the distributions of the estimators become more and more concentrated near the true value of the parameter being estimated, so that the probability of the estimator being arbitrarily close to the parameter converges to one. An estimator for a parameter is *consistent* if the estimator converges in probability to the true value of the parameter; that is, the limit in probability of the estimator, as the sample size goes to infinity, is the parameter itself (Fig. 6.1). In other words, an estimator is consistent if it has an asymptotic power of one (Parson, *Illustrated Dictionary of Economics,* p. 47).

An *efficient estimator* is an estimator that estimates the parameter of interest with the smallest variance. In other words, it has minimum variance among estimates of its kind.

Missing completely at random (MCAR) refers to missing observations, but the way they are missing does not depend on observed or unobserved measurements. Some refer to this sample as *uniform nonresponse*. The key fact is that we expect

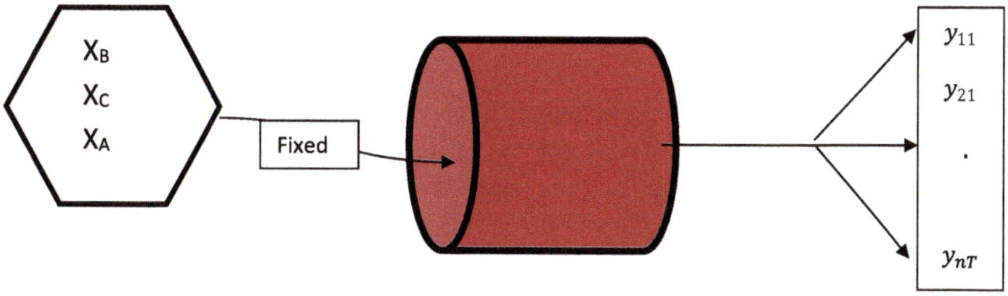

Fig. 6.1 Depicting GEE logistic regression model

consistent results with missing data. Of course, there is generally be some loss of information. However, in practice, MCAR means that the analysis of only those units with complete data can provide the opportunity for valid inferences. An example of this phenomenon would be if one of the patients from the study dies in a car accident, there is no information about this patient that are used to conduct the study and analyze the data. We do not see anything based on the data collected that would lead to the accident, and the patient's data can no longer be used in analysis because the patient cannot be rehospitalized.

The *score function* is a weighted product of the information from the covariate and the residual. When this function is set to zero, we obtain the estimates of the regression coefficient in the systematic component. In a repeated data setting, the repeats for an individual are connected through a so-called working covariance matrix. This is similar in form to the estimating equation (called normal equations when dealing with standard normal regression models) for β in the well-known normal model. Upon convergence, standard errors associated with β are obtained as the square root of the diagonal elements of the information matrix (Gibbons & Hedeker, 1997).

Information matrix or the observed information, or observed Fisher information, is the negative of the second derivative (the Hessian matrix) of the "log likelihood" (the logarithm of the likelihood function). It is important to obtaining the variance of the estimator.

Information criteria provide a measure of the information lost by considering a model in place of the raw data, so smaller values of information criteria suggest better fit.

Estimating equations is a relationship involving the parameters of a statistical model, thereby leading to a method of estimation.

Working correlation matrix is usually unknown and must be estimated. It provides weights for the combination of the correlated responses as the regression coefficients are estimated.

Marginal models are used to demonstrate that the model for the mean response at each occasion depends only on the covariates of interest, and not on any random effects or previous responses.

Wald confidence intervals are sometimes called the normal confidence intervals. They are based on the asymptotic normality of the parameter estimators and obtained by taking the estimator, plus or minus the reliability coefficient times the standard error.

6.3 Exploratory Analyses

Correlated outcomes are encountered in many areas of research and occur for a variety of reasons. Valid statistical inferences require that we properly account for the correlation among outcomes within subjects. Ignoring the correlation will likely lead to an underestimation of the variance. This type of within-subject correlation is due to a single outcome measured repeatedly over time on the same subject, as in longitudinal studies and in the *Medicare* data, or may be due to multiple outcomes measured one or more times, each on the same subject, as in clinical trials involving multiple endpoints. Correlation may also be due to a commonality related to output among units (families or litters) which is the case in so-called clustered data.

For example, there is a sample of 1625 patients in the Medicare dataset with complete information; each has three outcomes indicating the different times he/she was rehospitalized. Though there are methods for dealing with unbalanced data, this chapter only considers those subjects who have complete data at all 3 consecutive time points, resulting in 1625 subjects with 3 observations for each. Table 6.1 shows some lines of that data.

The standard logistic regression model (Chap. 3) addresses the odds, and, as such, the parameters are readily interpretable. The standard logistic regression model relies on the assumption that the observations are independent; thus, they are not utilized as we have correlated observations. Our interests lie in the cases or situations when the observations are not independent. For example,

- Subjects are followed; the covariates and responses are repeatedly measured.
- Subjects/units exist in a cluster or family or group.
- Subjects/units provide several responses over time.
- Subjects/units are treated under different experimental conditions.

Figure 6.1 presents the structure as deemed useful for GEE logistic regression models. The responses are correlated as they are produced and reproduced by the same mechanism. These unit outcomes are denoted by y_{1j}, y_{2j}, ...y_{nj}. where y_{ij} represents the *j*th measure on the *i*th unit. The covariates X_B, X_A, X_C represent the input variables, which are considered to be fixed for each individual. These can be categorical X_A, binary X_B, or continuous X_C.

Assumption The model assumes that the units $y_{ij}$are independent though the y_{ij} and y_{st} are not when *i* and *s* are equal. The outcomes are binary. In other words, units within a cluster are correlated, but units across clusters are independent. There are two basic approaches for modeling binary responses that account for correlation:

1. The marginal model addresses the autocorrelation through the random component, where we address the distribution of the responses.
2. The subject specific model assumes that there is a natural heterogeneity due to the random effects. This heterogeneity can be modeled by a probability distribution and is addressed in the systematic component, where we talk about the covariates that are included in the model. We concentrate on approach 1 in this chapter.

Table 6.1 Partial data in the Medicare data as used for analysis

PNUM_R	biRadmit	NDX	NPR	LOS	DX101	Time
127	0	9	6	6	1	1
127	0	6	4	1	1	2
127	0	9	5	3	1	3
560	1	9	3	8	0	1
560	0	9	1	17	0	2
560	0	7	1	6	0	3
746	1	6	4	12	0	1
746	0	6	1	1	0	2
746	0	9	1	2	0	3
750	0	9	3	6	0	1
750	1	7	3	4	0	2
750	1	9	2	4	0	3
1568	1	8	1	2	0	1
1568	1	9	1	4	0	2
1568	0	8	3	2	0	3
2076	1	9	5	8	1	1
2076	0	9	6	17	0	2
2076	1	9	1	6	0	3
2390	0	7	2	2	0	1
2390	0	7	2	3	0	2
2390	0	5	1	3	0	3
2413	0	9	6	17	0	1
2413	0	8	3	9	1	2

We present a GEE logistic regression model for analyzing these binary data because GEE models are useful for situations when the data are correlated. They are also useful when the sampling units are repeatedly measured. GEE logistic models allow missing completely at random (MCAR) values within a subject without losing all the data from that subject. It also allows time-dependent predictors in the model. However, the GEE model requires a large number of subjects and takes into consideration autocorrelation in the responses. Such correlation is addressed in the random component of the generalized linear model setup of random, systematic, and link components. It is a population-averaged model. However, since the distribution of the repeated observations is unknown, we cannot use the maximum likelihood method (Zeger & Liang, 1986a, b).

GEEs were developed as a means of analyzing longitudinal data when correlation is present (Breslow, 1989; Davidian & Carroll, 1987). The presence of correlation makes it impossible to write down the joint likelihood; thus, a quasi-likelihood-based approach for modeling correlated responses is used. We are unable to present the likelihood due to the nonindependence, thereby losing the opportunity to use the product of the probabilities to obtain the likelihood.

The GEE procedure extends the generalized linear model to allow for the analysis of repeated measurements or other correlated observations, such as clustered data. The GEE approach of Zeger and Liang facilitates the analysis of data collected in longitudinal, nested, or repeated measures designs. Though the specification of a working correlation matrix accounts for the form of within-subject correlation of responses, GEEs provide more efficient and unbiased regression parameters relative to ordinary least squares. The individual response may come from one of many distributions, including binomial and Poisson (Ballinger, 2004). It is the joint distribution of the repeats that necessitates the GEE approximations.

The true distribution of responses does not necessarily have to be specified for estimating the regression coefficients. We just need to specify a mean-variance relation. As GEE models are based on "quasi-likelihood" methods, the joint distribution of a subject's responses does not need to be specified. We only need the marginal distribution of a subject's response y_{11} at each time point. Thus, GEE models avoid the need to specify the joint distributions for binary longitudinal data. If we are to use the standard logistic regression model, we will get the following results.

Response Profile

Ordered value	biRadmit	Total frequency
1	0	2433
2	1	2442

Probability modeled is biRadmit = 1

It treats the 4875 observations as though they are independent. So, they can use the log likelihood to obtain the *analysis of maximum likelihood estimates* with the following results:

Parameter	DF	Estimate	Standard Error	Chi-Square	Wald Pr > ChiSq
Intercept	1	-0.3675	0.1263	8.4600	0.0036
NDX	1	0.0648	0.0154	17.6382	<.0001
NPR	1	-0.0306	0.0186	2.7115	0.0996
LOS	1	0.0344	0.00555	38.4549	<.0001
DX101	1	-0.1143	0.0913	1.5667	0.2107
T2	1	-0.3876	0.0716	29.2711	<.0001
T3	1	-0.2412	0.0721	11.1925	0.0008

Odds Ratio Estimates

Effect	Point Estimate	95% Wald Confidence Limits	
NDX	1.067	1.035	1.100
NPR	0.970	0.935	1.006
LOS	1.035	1.024	1.046
DX101	0.892	0.746	1.067
T2	0.679	0.590	0.781
T3	0.786	0.682	0.905

Using the standard logistic regression model suggests that NDX ($p < 0.0001$), LOS (<0.0001), and time (<0.0001) were significant. However, it makes no allowances for the fact that responses on a patient are correlated.

6.4 Statistical Models: GEE Logistic Regression

6.4.1 Medicare Data

We fit several different GEE logistic regression models where the estimates depend on the covariance structure. Let us consider independence, compound symmetry, autoregressive (AR (1)), unstructured, and user-defined working correlation structures, but the possibilities are not limited to these familiar relations.

6.4.2 Generalized Linear Model

The generalized linear model (Chap. 3) provides a framework for modeling continuous response by extending traditional linear model theory to non-normal data. In cross-sectional studies, each subject has a single observation, and a generalized linear model (McCullagh & Nelder, 1989) is used to regress a variety of covariates. However, since GLMs assume that all observations are independent of each other, they are not appropriate for the analysis of longitudinal data. Moreover, in studies, such as prospective cohort studies, where individuals are observed for multiple occurrences, the outcomes are often correlated. Such correlation is treated with statistical consideration by including the repeated measures. In such cases, the generalized estimating equations can be used to analyze the data with reasonable statistical efficiency (Ziang & Leger, 1986a, b). However, in those cases, when the observations are correlated, we cannot readily obtain the underlying joint distribution; hence, there is no closed-form joint likelihood function to present, as is the case with the standard logistic regression model. One remedy for modeling the correlated observations is to fit a GEE logistic regression model. We fit such types of correlated models in this chapter and present alternative approaches in Chaps. 7 and 8.

6.4.3 Generalized Estimating Equations

When the effects of the covariates on the outcome variable are the primary focus, the generalized estimating equation (GEE) model is an extension of generalized linear models as applied to the analysis of longitudinal data (Liang & Zeger, 1986). The GEE model is an extension of the GLM to correlated data. The components (random, systematic, and link) in the GEE are defined similar to what is done with the GLM. Instead of a random component providing full information on the distribution, there is limited information. The systematic and link functions provide information as they did in GLM. So, for example, the linear predictor for a GEE logistic regression model with two covariates is given with its systematic and logit link functions as

$$\eta_t = \beta_0 + \beta_1 X_{1t} + \beta_2 X_{2t}$$

$$\eta_t = \log\left[p_{1t}/p_{0t}\right]$$

where X_{1t} and X_{2t} are two covariates for subject *i* at time *t*, with a logit link function.

Liang and Zeger developed the GEE models (Liang & Zeger, 1986; Zeger & Liang, 1986a, b). In the GEE model, there is no defined likelihood and hence there are no maximum likelihood estimates, but there are quasi-likelihood estimates for the coefficients. These estimates are obtained from the quasi-score function. So, a GLM comes with systematic and link functions and a fully described distribution, while a GEE has link and systematic functions, but the distributional assumption is based only on the mean and variance relation.

When GEE logistic regression models consider a given subject as measured at all T time points, then it is the full $T \times T$ correlation matrix of the longitudinal data to which we refer. It is the average over all the observations and hence the reason that GEE accommodates missing data on a subject. So, if the largest number of repeats on a subject is three but one subject only has two repeats, then we present a matrix of the larger dimension of 3.

6.4.4 Marginal Model

The GEE logistic regression models are considered marginal models since they seek to characterize the expectation of a subject's response y at time t as a function of the subject's covariates at time t. As a marginal model, the GEE model is appropriate when inferences about the population average is of primary interest (Diggle et al., 1994) or when the expectation of the response variable is being regressed on some function of covariates in order to make future applications with the results (Pepe & Anderson, 1994).

Marginal models assume that repeated observations from the same subject are generally correlated. Thus, for a particular time t, the marginal density of y_{it} is assumed to follow a generalized linear model (McCullagh & Nelder, 1989) with the random distribution of the outcome values belonging to the exponential family. The regression of the response on explanatory variables is modeled separately from the within-person correlation. We model the mean of the response over the subpopulation sharing a common value of the covariates, and interpretation relates to the population and not the individual (Hu et al., 1998).

6.4.5 Working Correlation Matrices

The GEE models consist of a matrix referred to as the *working correlation matrix* representing the structure of the repeated measures on a subject. This matrix includes the assumption made regarding the association between the observations for each subject. In fitting the model, we assume that the form of the relation, and not necessarily the degree of that relation, is the same for all subjects. Therefore, if we assume that there is compound symmetry for one subject, we assume this is true for all subjects. In reality, however, even if the structure is the same, the strength of that association may differ across subjects. Thus, the model takes the average across all subjects and uses that as the correlation. The typical working correlations for GEE models are independence, compound symmetry or exchangeability, autoregressive AR (1), unstructured, and user-defined correlation structure:

- *Independence* indicates that repeated observations are uncorrelated. It is the simplest form of working correlation, namely, the identity matrix of dimension T. This form indicates that the longitudinal data are not correlated. In general, this is not intuitive and would be difficult to accept. However, Pepe and Anderson (1994) indicate that use of the independence structure does have certain advantages if the models include time-dependent covariates (Chap. 7).
- *Exchangeable* indicates correlation between any two responses if the ith subject/unit is the same. The exchangeable or compound-symmetry correlation assumes that all of the correlations are the same. So, if a subject is measured four times, then correlation of observations at times (1, 2), (1, 3), (1, 4), (2, 3), (2, 4), and (3, 4) are all the same.

- *Autoregressive (AR (1))* indicates another useful correlation for longitudinal data. It tells us that the correlation between any two observations is assumed to be less as they become further apart and is measured by $\rho^{\{\text{time period difference}\}}$. Since it depends only on one parameter term, it is very parsimonious for longitudinal data. This autoregressive assumption (also referred to as a "transitional model") is used when the analysis must account for a time dependency.
- *Unstructured* or unspecified indicates that the correlation within any two responses is unknown and must be estimated. Thus, no structural form is assumed, and it may be that all correlations per subject/unit are different. This unstructured form is the most efficient but is only useful if the numbers of time points are small; otherwise, there are too many parameters to be estimated.
- *User-defined* structure indicates that the analyst decides (maybe from past studies or experience) what the correlations at any two responses ought to be. This choice for working correlation is not well-advised since it can lead to non-convergence.

Modeling the correlation with the GEE approach accounts for the association across time and the association between observations for the same subject. As such, it allows an arbitrary working correlation structure for the correlation matrix of a subject's outcomes. We present an average of these correlation matrices.

6.4.6 Model Fit

When fitting the standard logistic regression, the appropriateness of the fit is measured since we have likelihoods and joint likelihoods on account of the independent observations with known distribution. However, the fit of GEE logistic regression model cannot be assessed in such a manner because of the lack of independence with correlated observations. The most common fit statistic for the GEE logistic regression model is the quasi-likelihood information criterion, or QIC (Pan & Connett, 2002). QIC is used to compare models with different working correlation structures, where the model with the smallest QIC is selected. QIC is used to select among models with different combinations of predictors.

6.4.7 Properties of GEE Estimates

It is natural to question how these estimates in a GEE logistic regression model perform. The regression coefficient estimators in the GEE models have the following properties:

1. They are consistent and asymptotically normal even with misspecification of the correlation structure (Liang & Zeger, 1986). That is appealing since one may not always select the corrected correlation matrix.

2. The standard errors can be consistently estimated regardless of whether or not the working correlation structure is correctly specified.
3. However, their efficiency is reduced if the choice of correlation matrix is incorrect; and the loss of efficiency gets small as the number of subjects gets large (Zeger & Liang, 1992).

The GEE logistic regression model is best suited for scenarios with only a few time points and when each subject has complete data with a good choice of the working correlation matrix (Diggle et al., 1994).

6.5 Data Analysis

6.5.1 GEE Logistic Regression Model

We fit GEE logistic regression models to the Medicare data using SAS, SPSS, R, and STATA for the analysis of the probability of rehospitalization. These models adjust for the correlation through the random component. We fitted the logistic regression model:

$$\log\left(P_{y=1} | P_{y=0}\right) = \beta_0 + \beta_1 \text{NDX} + \beta_2 \text{NPR} + \beta_3 \text{LOS} + \beta_4 \text{DX101} + \beta_5 T_2 + \beta_6 T_3$$

with several working correlation structures where $P_{y=1}$ denotes the probability of rehospitalization within 30 days, $P_{y=0}$ denotes the probability of not being rehospitalized within 30 days, NDX denotes the total number of diagnoses, NPR denotes the number of prescriptions, LOS denotes the length of stay, DX101 is binary and denotes the presence of coronary atherosclerosis, T_2 denotes period 2, and T_3 denotes period 3. We fit each of the working correlation matrices: independence, compound symmetry, autoregressive, unstructured, and user-defined. We used SAS, SPSS, R, and STATA.

6.5.2 GEE Logistic Regression Model with SAS Programming

SAS Program

```
data mydata; set chapter6;
T2=(time=2); T3=(time=3); run;
title 'GEE with AR(1) corr structure';
proc genmod data=mydata descend; * to model Prob(y=1);
class PNUM_R time;
model biRadmit=NDX NPR LOS DX101 T2 T3 / dist=BIN;
repeated subject=PNUM_R /within=time corr=AR(1) corrw;
output out=GEEout xbeta=xb RESRAW = rraw;
run;
```

Comment biRadmit denotes the binary outcome; PNUM_R denotes the patient ID. This identifies the cluster and in this case the patient is the cluster (of size 3 in this case); CORR = AR (1) signifies to SAS to use the autoregressive working correlation structure order 1. Other working structures can be used by using the appropriate name. The program runs the GEE model with working correlation structure. The repeat (cluster) is identified by SUBJECT=. The program inherently assumes that the data have been saved in "long" format, meaning each observation time for each individual corresponds to a unique row in the dataset. The working correlation is invoked with the WITHIN = time CORR = AR (1). OUT is a SAS word. GEEout is our name for the dataset with the results of the predicted probabilities in xbeta (=$\beta_0 + \beta_1$NDX + β_2NPR + β_3LOS + β_4DX101 + $\beta_5 T_2 + \beta_6 T_3$), and the raw residuals are in RESRAW (=observed- predicted).

Comment OUT is a SAS word. GEEout is our name for the dataset with the results of the predicted logits in xbeta, and the raw residuals are RESRAW.

SAS Output

```
                    GEE with AR (1) corr structure
                         The GENMOD Procedure
                          Model Information
Data Set                                                   WORK.MYDATA
Distribution                                               Binomial
Link Function                                              Logit
Dependent Variable          biRadmit                       biRadmit
Number of Observations Read                                4875
Number of Observations Used                                4875
Number of Events                                           2442
Number of Trials                                           4875
```

Comment There are 4875 data points because the analysis is looking at the results of 1625 patients with 3 measures each (1625 × 3 = 4875).

```
                         Class Level Information
          Class        Levels     Values
PNUM_R    1625    127 560 746 750 1117 1395 1568 2076 2390 2413 3008
3123 3710 3970 3982 4236 4581 4873 5387 6255 7497
7599 8181 9677 10464 11050 11274 11279 11787 13420
13436 13761 14955 16160 16464 16971 17748 18638
18697 19349 19674 19730 20112 20973 21410 21800
...
time                3    1 2 3
```

Comment There are 3 time points and the 1625 patients are presented with their ID numbers. We truncated the list of class levels for space reasons, but the program will list all.

Response Profile

```
Response Profile
Ordered                    bi                  Total
Value                      Radmit              Frequency
1                          1                   2442
2                          0                   2433
PROC GENMOD is modeling the probability that biRadmit='1'.
```

Comment GENMOD is modeling log [(Prob Radmit =1)/(Prob Radmit =0)]. Adding the numbers in the total frequency column shows that we have the correct amount of total data points (2442 + 2433 = 4875 = 1625 × 3).

```
                      Parameter Information
Parameter            Effect
Prm1                 Intercept
Prm2                 NDX
Prm3                 NPR
Prm4                 LOS
Prm5                 DX101
Prm6                 T2
Prm7                 T3
```

Comment These are the parameters in the model presented to SAS to run:

$$\log\left(P_{y=1}|P_{y=0}\right)=\beta_0+\beta_1\text{NDX}+\beta_2\text{NPR}+\beta_3\text{LOS}+\beta_4\text{DX101}+\beta_5T_2+\beta_6T_3$$

```
                      The GENMOD Procedure
                      Algorithm converged.
                      GEE Model Information
Correlation Structure                              AR (1)
Within-Subject Effect                        time (3 levels)
Subject Effect                         PNUM_R (1625 levels)
Number of Clusters                                  1625
Correlation Matrix Dimension                        3
Maximum Cluster Size                                3
Minimum Cluster Size                                3
                      Algorithm converged.
```

Comment The AR (1) model is autoregressive. There are three points (times) in each cluster. The program converged. They do not always.

Working Correlation Matrix

	Col1	Col2	Col3
Row1	1.0000	0.0294	0.0009
Row2	0.0294	1.0000	0.0294
Row3	0.0009	0.0294	1.0000

Comment The working correlation matrix is the AR (1) = the autoregressive of order 1. Note that (Row1, Col2) = (Row2, Col3) = (Row2, Col1) = (Row3, Col2) =0.0294. Responses from observation times that differ by 1 are equally correlated. Similarly (Row1, Col3) = (Row3, Col1) =0.0009 = $(0.0294)^2$. The autocorrelation is squared to correspond to responses taken two periods away. Responses from observation times differing by 2 are equally correlated.

GEE Fit Criteria

QIC	6648.5528
QICu	6646.6229

Comment This is a measure of the fit of the model. However, since there is no declared distribution, one has nothing to compare it to. You can, however, use it to compare nested models.

Analysis Of GEE Parameter Estimates
Empirical Standard Error Estimates

Parameter	Estimate	Standard Error	95% Confidence Limits		Z	Pr > |Z|
Intercept	-0.3614	0.1258	-0.6079	-0.1148	-2.87	0.0041
NDX	0.0645	0.0160	0.0331	0.0958	4.03	<.0001
NPR	-0.0290	0.0191	-0.0665	0.0084	-1.52	0.1282
LOS	0.0331	0.0076	0.0182	0.0481	4.35	<.0001
DX101	-0.1239	0.0936	-0.3073	0.0595	-1.32	0.1854
T2	-0.3865	0.0710	-0.5258	-0.2473	-5.44	<.0001
T3	-0.2401	0.0688	-0.3750	-0.1053	-3.49	0.0005

Comment The fitted logistic regression model is

$$\log\left[\frac{P_1}{P_0}\right] = -0.361 + 0.065\text{NDX} - 0.029\text{NPR} + 0.033\text{LOS} - 0.124\text{DX101}$$
$$-0.387\text{T}_2 - 0.240\text{T}_3$$

The variables NDX ($p < 0.001$) and LOS ($p < 0.001$), as well as T_2 and T_3 , are significant.

We present the results from some other working correlation matrices. We chose only to include the outputs as they pertained to the coefficients and the working matrix.

6.5.3 GEE Logistic Regression Model with SPSS Programming

We used SPSS to fit the GEE logistic regression models.

SPSS Program

```
                    SPSS Pull Down Menu
Step 1:
In the data editor window select "Variable View" in the bottom
left corner
Make sure the following variables are set to the following
"Measure"
1) PNUM_R → Scale
2) biRadmit → Nominal
3) NDX → Scale
4) NPR → Scale
5) LOS → Scale
6) DX101 → Scale
7) T2 → Nominal
8) T3 → Nominal
STEP 2:
Click "Analyze" on the toolbar
Select "Generalized Linear Models"
Click "Generalized Estimating Equations"
STEP 3:
Click the first tab labeled "Repeated"
Select the subject variable in the left column
Click the arrow next to "Subject variables:"
Select the Within-subject variable in the left column
Click the arrow next to "Within-subject variables:"
Click the box next to "Structure:" under "Working
Correlation Matrix"
Select "Exchangeable", "Independent", "AR (1)", or "Unstructured"
accordingly
```

```
STEP 4:
Click the second tab labeled "Type of Model"
Select "Binary logistic" under "Binary Response or Events/
Trials Data"
Step 5:
Click the third tab labeled "Response"
Select the Dependent variable in the left column
Click the arrow next to "Dependent Variable"
Step 6:
Click the third tab labeled "Predictors"
Select the Independent variables in the left column
Click the arrow next to "Covariates:"
Step 7:
Click the fourth tab labeled "Model"
Select the Independent variables in the left column
Click the arrow under "Build Term(s)"
Click "OK" at the bottom of the window
```

If we were to use the corrtype = auto regressive, we will get the following:

Parameter Estimates for Autoregressive Working Correlation

			95% Wald confidence interval		Hypothesis test		Hypothesis test
Parameter	B	Std. error	Lower	Upper	Wald chi-square	DF	Sig.
(Intercept)	0.387	0.1255	0.141	0.633	9.529	1	0.002
NDX	−0.069	0.0160	−0.100	−0.037	18.475	1	0.000
NPR	0.027	0.0190	−0.010	0.064	2.041	1	0.153
LOS	−0.031	0.0075	−0.046	−0.017	17.513	1	0.000
DX101	0.126	0.0934	−0.057	0.309	1.822	1	0.177
T2	0.387	0.0710	0.248	0.526	29.691	1	0.000
T3	0.239	0.0688	0.104	0.374	12.066	1	0.001
(Scale)	1						

Comment For the AR (1) working correlation matrix, we use CORRTYPE = AR (1) in the code or choose the AR (1) option in the pull-down menu. The information obtained from the output is similar on the correlation defined but for the parameter estimates standard error. Then the fitted model is

$$\log\left[\frac{P_1}{P_0}\right] = 0.387 - 0.069\mathrm{NDX} + 0.027\mathrm{NPR} - 0.031\mathrm{LOS}$$
$$+ 0.126\mathrm{DX101} + 0.387\mathrm{T}_2 + 0.239\mathrm{T}_3$$

AR (1) says that the correlation at adjacent times when squared is the same between two time periods apart.

Parameter Estimates for AR (1) Working Correlation

			95% Wald confidence interval		Hypothesis test		Hypothesis test
Parameter	B	Std. error	Lower	Upper	Wald chi-square	DF	Sig.
(Intercept)	0.361	0.1258	0.115	0.608	8.253	1	0.004
NDX	−0.064	0.0160	−0.096	−0.033	16.265	1	0.000
NPR	0.029	0.0191	−0.008	0.066	2.315	1	0.128
LOS	−0.033	0.0076	−0.048	−0.018	18.958	1	0.000
DX101	0.124	0.0936	−0.059	0.307	1.754	1	0.185
T2	0.387	0.0710	0.247	0.526	29.617	1	0.000
T3	0.240	0.0688	0.105	0.375	12.187	1	0.000
(Scale)	1						

Comment The fitted model is

$$\log\left[\frac{P_1}{P_0}\right] = 0.361 - 0.064\text{NDX} + 0.029\text{NPR} - 0.033\text{LOS}$$
$$+ 0.124\text{DX101} + 0.387\text{T}_2 + 0.240\text{T}_3$$

We fitted the GEE logistic regression models with R. NDX, LOS, and time are all significant in the model.

6.5.4 GEE Logistic Regression Model with R Programming

R Program

```
> geeglm.out=geeglm(formula = biRadmit ~ NDX + NPR + LOS + DX101
+ T2 + T3, data=chapter6, family=binomial, corstr="ar1",
id=PNUM_R)
> summary(geeglm.out)
Call:
geeglm(formula = biRadmit ~ NDX + NPR + LOS + DX101 + T2 + T3,
 family = binomial, data = chapter6, id = PNUM_R, corstr = "ar1")
```

Comment Family = Binomial refers to the distribution assumed for the outcomes in a certain year. The corstr = "ar1" determines the autoregressive (1) working correlation matrix structure.

R Output

```
Coefficients:
              Estimate    Std.err         Wald       Pr(>|W|)
(Intercept)   -0.3607     0.1258          8.22       0.00414 **
NDX             0.0644    0.0160         16.25       5.6e-05 ***
NPR           -0.0289     0.0191          2.29       0.13039
LOS             0.0330    0.0076         18.84       1.4e-05 ***
DX101         -0.1250     0.0936          1.78       0.18174
T2            -0.3864     0.0710         29.60       5.3e-08 ***
T3            -0.2400     0.0688         12.18       0.00048 ***
Signif. codes:  0 '***' 0.001 '**' 0.01 '*' 0.05 '.' 0.1 ' ' 1

Estimated Scale Parameters:
             Estimate Std.err
(Intercept)      1.02   0.259
Correlation: Structure = ar1 Link = identity
Estimated Correlation Parameters:
Estimate Std.err
alpha   0.0326 0.0192
Number of clusters:   1625   Maximum cluster size: 3
```

Comment The fitted logistic regression model is

$$\log\left[\frac{P_1}{P_0}\right] = -0.361 + 0.064\text{NDX} - 0.029\text{NPR} + 0.033\text{LOS}$$
$$- 0.125\text{DX101} - 0.386\text{T}_2 - 0.240\text{T}_3$$

NDX, LOS, and time are significant factors in rehospitalization. The correlation is 0.0326 with a standard error of 0.0192.

6.5.5 *GEE Logistic Regression Model with STATA Programming*

```
. xtgee biRadmit NDX NPR LOS DX101 T2   T3, family(binomial 1)
link(logit) corr(ar 1)
Iteration 1:   Tolerance = .00816804
Iteration 2:   Tolerance = .00030486
Iteration 3:   Tolerance = .00001228
Iteration 4:   Tolerance = 5.405e-07
```

```
GEE population-averaged model              Number of obs      =   4,875
Group and time vars: PNUM_R tim            Number of groups   =   1,625
Family: Binomial                           Obs per group:
Link:    Logit                                          min   =       3
Correlation: AR(1)                                      avg   =     3.0
                                                        max   =       3
                                           Wald chi2(6)       =  112.54
Scale parameter = 1                        Prob > chi2        =  0.0000
```

biRadmit	Coefficient	Std. err.	z	P>z	[95% conf.	interval]
NDX	.0645791	.0154795	4.17	0.000	.0342398	.0949185
NPR	-.0293369	.018626	-1.58	0.115	-.0658431	.0071694
LOS	.0331965	.0055376	5.99	0.000	.022343	.04405
DX101	-.1200396	.091516	-1.31	0.190	-.2994076	.0593285
T2	-.3865062	.0705882	-5.48	0.000	-.5248566	-.2481559
T3	-.2400372	.0720502	-3.33	0.001	-.381253	-.0988214
_cons	-.3622275	.1267884	-2.86	0.004	-.6107281	-.1137269

Comment For the AR (1) working correlation matrix, we use CORRTYPE = AR (1) in the code or choose the AR (1) option in the pull-down menu. The information on the output is similar but for the parameter estimates. Then the fitted model is

$$\log\left[\frac{P_1}{P_0}\right] = 0.387 - 0.065\text{NDX} + 0.027\text{NPR} - 0.031\text{LOS}$$
$$+ 0.126\text{DX101} + 0.387\text{T}_2 + 0.239\text{T}_3$$

AR (1) says that the correlation between adjacent time when squared is the correlation between events time periods apart.

6.6 Conclusion

There are repeated measurements on the rehospitalization of the patient as well as patients' lengths of stay, numbers of diagnoses, and others as covariates. These are correlated observations. In analyzing these data, we demonstrate the fit of GEE models to *Medicare* data using SAS, SPSS, R, and STATA. The GEE logistic regression models are fitted to correlated data using generalized estimating equations. The approach with this model, when accounting for the dependency in the data, is to treat the correlation as a nuisance. In particular, the correlation is addressed by assuming certain assumptions about the association among the observations. In practice, it addresses the problem through the random component of the model. The

Table 6.2 Estimates and standard errors for GEE logistic regression models

	Independence	Symmetry	Autoregressive	Unstructured	User-defined
Parameter	Est./std. err	Est./std. err	Est./std. err	Est./std. err	Est./std. err
Intercept	−0.368/0.126	−0.371/0.126	−0.361/0.126	−0.387/0.126	−0.045/0.212
NDX	**0.065/0.016**	**0.066/0.016**	**0.065/0.016**	**0.069/0.016**	0.029/0.028
NPR	−0.030/0.019	−0.027/0.019	−0.029/0.019	−0.027/0.019	0.033/0.030
LOS	**0.034/0.008**	0.031/0.008	**0.033/0.008**	**0.031/0.008**	−0.003/0.009
DX101	−0.114/0.094	−0.133/0.093	−0.123/0.094	−0.126/0.093	**−0.364/0.158**
T2	**−0.388/0.071**	**−0.386/0.071**	**−0.387/0.071**	**−0.387/0.071**	**−0.353/0.071**
T3	**−0.241/0.069**	**−0.239/0.069**	**−0.240/0.069**	**−0.239/0.069**	**−0.191/0.071**

GEE logistic regression models are fitted to the rehospitalization data using five different (independence, exchangeability, autoregressive, unstructured, and user-defined) working correlation matrices. As the subjects are repeatedly measured, we expect inherent correlation among the responses per subject. The results pertaining to the predictors, NDX, NPR, LOS, and DX101, are similar in four of the five cases. A summary of the results is given in Table 6.1. From Table 6.1, we see that NDX and LOS are significant in all four cases where the data determine the estimates of the correlation. This is not the case when a user-defined working correlation matrix is given with no information from the data. Though this is not a simulation study, it is useful to note that standard errors are larger for user-defined matrices than any of the other type of working matrices. Also, the results for the dummy variables T2 and T3 (indicating the period of rehospitalization) are identical regardless of the working correlation matrix chosen. This is to be expected as we are fitting main effects models. Because the GEE logistic regression model is a population-averaged or marginal model, the parameter estimates describe expected differences in the mean response between populations that differed according to values of the predictors.

These parameter estimates do not allow us to make conclusions about changing values for individuals. The parameter results are similar, except those for the user-defined matrix. The user-defined working correlation matrix gives conflicting results. This contradiction reminds us that while GEE is a viable resource, the prescribed covariance matrix cannot be arbitrary, and otherwise the predictors have values assumed to be what they are not. These GEE models assume that the covariates are time-independent. The models do not take into account the fact that these covariates are time-dependent. In Chap. 7, we revisit these data and take into account the time-dependent covariates (Table 6.2).

6.7 Related Examples

The 1980 National Center for Education Statistics' National Longitudinal Survey, "High School and Beyond," has, among other things, the aspirations regarding college question that was asked at each wave (Wilson & Wilson, 1992). One can find the sample design, sample selection, and sample results at http://eric.ed.

gov/?id = ED214990 in Chap. 2, where it discusses the construction of the sample frame of high schools in the United States. Chapter 3 presented the frame with respect to its stratified design, while the actual school selection procedures and results are reviewed in Chap. 4. Chapter 5 then describes the construction of the student sampling frame, the selection of students, and certain results. The survey design included a highly stratified national probability sample of 1106 secondary schools as the first-stage units of selection. In the second stage, 36 seniors and 36 sophomores were selected per school. Sampling rates for each stratum were set so as to select in each stratum the number of schools needed to satisfy study design criteria regarding minimum sample sizes for certain types of schools. One can fit a GEE logistic regression model to determine the baseline characteristics that may influence their aspirations to go to college over time.

References

Ballinger, G. A. (2004). Using generalized estimating equations for longitudinal data analysis. *Organizational Research Methods, 7*, 127–150.

Breslow, N. E. (1989). Score tests in overdispersed GLMs. In A. Decarli, B. J. Francis, R. Gilchrist, & G. U. H. Seeber (Eds.), *Workshop on statistical Modeling* (pp. 64–74). Springer-Verlag.

Davidian, M., & Carroll, R. J. (1987). Variance function estimation. *Journal ofAmerican Statistical Association, 82*, 1079–1091.

Diggle, P. J., Liang, K. Y., & Zeger, S. L. (1994). *Analysis of longitudinal data.* Oxford University Press.

Galbraith, S., Daniel, J. A., & Vissel, B. (2010). A study of clustered data and approaches to its analysis. *Journal of Neuroscience, 30*, 10601–10608.

Gibbons, R. D., & Hedeker, D. H. (1997). Random effects probit and logistic regression models for three-level data. *Biometrics, 53*, 1527–1537.

Hardin, J. W., & Hilbe, J. M. (2003). *Generalized estimating equations*. Wiley.

Hu, F. B., Goldberg, J., Hedeker, D., Flay, B. R., & Pentz, M. A. (1998). Comparison of population-averaged and subject-specific approaches for analyzing repeated binary outcomes. *American Journal of Epidemiology, 147*(7), 694–703.

Liang, K. Y., & Zeger, S. L. (1986). Longitudinal data analysis using generalized linear models. *Biometrika, 73*(1), 13–22.

McCullagh, P., & Nelder, J. (1989). *Generalized linear models* (2nd ed.). London.

Pan, W., & Connett, J. E. (2002). Selecting the working correlation structure in generalized estimating equations with application to the lung health study. *Statistica Sinica, 12*(2), 475–490.

Pepe, M. S., & Anderson, G. L. (1994). A cautionary note on inference for marginal regression models with longitudinal data and general correlated response data. *Communications in Statistics-Simulation and Computation, 23*(4), 939–951.

Wilson, P. M., & Wilson, J. R. (1992). Environmental influences on adolescent educational aspirations: A logistic transform model. *Youth & Society, 24*(1), 52–70.

Zeger, S. L., & Liang, K. Y. (1986a). Longitudinal data analysis for discrete and continuous outcomes. *Biometrics, 42*, 121–130.

Zeger, S. L., & Liang, K. Y. (1986b). Longitudinal data analysis using generalized linear models. *Biometrics, 73*, 13–22.

Zeger, S. L., & Liang, K. Y. (1992). An overview of methods for the analysis of longitudinal data. *Statistics in Medicine., 11*(14–15), 1825–1839.

Chapter 7
Generalized Method of Moments Logistic Regression Model

7.1 Motivating Example

7.1.1 Description of the Case Study

Medicare is a social insurance program, administered by the US government. It provides health insurance coverage to people who are aged 65 and over or those who meet other special criteria. We use a subset of data obtained regarding patient information obtained from an Arizona hospital discharge database for 3 years covered over a period from 2003 to 2005. The dataset contained the information of patients who are admitted to a hospital four times. There were 1625 patients in the dataset with information for all variables; each had three observations indicating the three different times each person is rehospitalized after the first visit to the hospital. Our response variable classification is based on those who returned to the hospital within 30 days as one and those who did not return as zero. The covariates considered are multitude of diseases (NDX), number of procedures (NPR), length of stay (LOS), and coronary atherosclerosis (DX101) as time-dependent. Our interest lies in modeling the probability of rehospitalization by identifying factors that may have an impact on rehospitalization. Besides the usual relation of covariates on responses at a particular point, we propose that responses in a present time period will impact covariates in a future time period and covariates in a present time period will likewise impact responses in future time periods. The problem is that such predictors have an inherent correlation that is fully explored and factored into any covariance matrix that is necessary to obtain estimates of the regression coefficients. The repeated measures of rehospitalization lead to correlation which, if ignored, underestimates the standard errors.

J. R. Wilson et al., *Modeling Binary Correlated Responses*, ICSA Book Series in Statistics, https://doi.org/10.1007/978-3-031-62427-8_7

7.1.2 Study Hypotheses

In the present data, we have sampling units of patients and observational units corresponding to each time a patient is observed. The binary response as well as the covariate values changes over time. So, researchers might wonder how the time-dependent covariates impact future covariate values as well as the responses. More importantly, the researchers might want to know if NPR, NDX, and DX101 have a significant impact on rehospitalization and how the covariates impact change differently over time.

7.2 Definition and Notation

A sampling unit is an individual item in a sample. It is associated with some probability of selection and is used to help ensure that the process is random.

An *observational unit* is an entity in which the value or the measurement is taken or obtained. The observational unit is a realization of the sampling unit.

Moment conditions is a method used to estimate the parameters of a statistical model. The method is based on obtaining a set of simultaneous equations that connect the sample data, and the model parameters are solved, thereby obtaining estimates of the parameters. For example, $E\left(\overline{X}\right)=\mu$ gives a moment estimate as $\hat{\mu}=n^{-1}\sum_{i=1}^{n}X_i$.

Generalized method of moments (GMM) is an extension of moment condition for estimating parameters in statistical models. This method involves combining the moment conditions through a weighted matrix, functions of the model parameters, and the data are specified such that the expected value is zero when computed at the true values of the parameters.

The GMM estimators are known to be *consistent*, asymptotically normal, and *efficient* since they belong to a class of estimators that does not use any extra information, aside from the data contained in the moment conditions (Hansen, 1982).

The continuously updating generalized method of moments estimator (CUGMM) is, (Hansen et al., 1996): Instead of estimating in 2 (or more) steps, it is based on one-time optimization: Computing this estimator is ~~are~~ computationally cumbersome.

A *time-dependent covariate* is a regressor that changes over time. If the regressor does not change over time, we refer to it as a *time-independent covariate*.

A *consistent estimator* or asymptotically consistent estimator is an estimator having the property that, as the number of data points used increases indefinitely, the resulting sequence of estimates converges in probability to the parameter value. This means that the distribution of the estimates becomes more and more concentrated close to the true value of the parameter being estimated; hence, the probability of the estimator, being arbitrarily close to the parameter value, converges to one.

Efficiency is a term used in the comparison of various statistical procedures, and, in particular, it refers to an experimental design or a hypothesis testing procedure. Essentially, a more efficient estimator necessitates a smaller sample size than a less efficient one to achieve the same goal. Efficiencies are often defined using the variance or mean square error as the measure of desirability.

The *relative efficiency* of two estimators is the ratio of their efficiencies. The efficiencies and the relative efficiency of two estimators depend on the sample size available for the given estimators. The asymptotic relative efficiency is defined as the limit of the relative efficiencies as the sample size grows. It is a common measure of comparison.

The *eta measure* is a measure of correlation between a binary variable and an ordinal model. One variable is identified as the response and the other as the covariate. The value changes depending on which is the binary measure. As a descriptive index of strength of association between an experimental factor (main effect or interaction effect) and a dependent variable, classical eta-squared is defined as the proportion of total variation attributable to the factor, and it ranges in value from 0 to 1 (Cohen et al., 2003; Hays, 1994; Maxwell & Delaney, 2000).

7.3 Exploratory Analyses

Since the Medicare data is composed of patient information with three time points, suggesting that there are trends over time, it is natural to wonder if there is a pattern that could predict the responses based on future covariates. An exploratory analysis is summarized, Table 7.1, and was conducted with some simple statistical tests to observe the relation between variables. A similar analysis was done to see the impact of present covariates on future responses (Table 7.2). Table 7.1 provides the bivariate relationships and the *p*-values for those simple statistical tests.

Based on these results, it seems that whether or not a patient is rehospitalized in 30 days is a significant impact on his or her length of stay the next time hospitalized ($p = 0.000$). Similarly, in Table 7.2, NDX at the previous hospitalization (in period 1- NDX_1) has a significant impact on whether or not the patient was rehospitalized within 30 days in periods 2 and 3 (Admit_2 and Admit_3) with *p*-values 0.000 and 0.003, respectively. The exploratory analysis suggests that there are correlations that need to be accounted for.

Figure 7.1 depicts the different types of correlations one may encounter as data are collected where the responses and input variables have different values at each

Table 7.1 p-values for impact of response (admit) on covariates (NDX, LOS, and DX101)

	NDX_2	NDX_3	LOS_2	LOS_3	DX101_2	DX101_3
Admit_1	0.151	0.016	0.000	0.014	0.194	0.357
Admit_2	–	0.975	–	0.634	–	0.328

Table 7.2 p-values for impact of covariates (NDX, LOS, and DX101) on response (admit)

	Admit_2	Admit_3
NDX_1	0.000	0.003
NDX_2	–	0.721
LOS_1	0.000	0.000
LOS_2	–	0.404
DX101_1	0.179	0.008
DX101_2	–	0.900

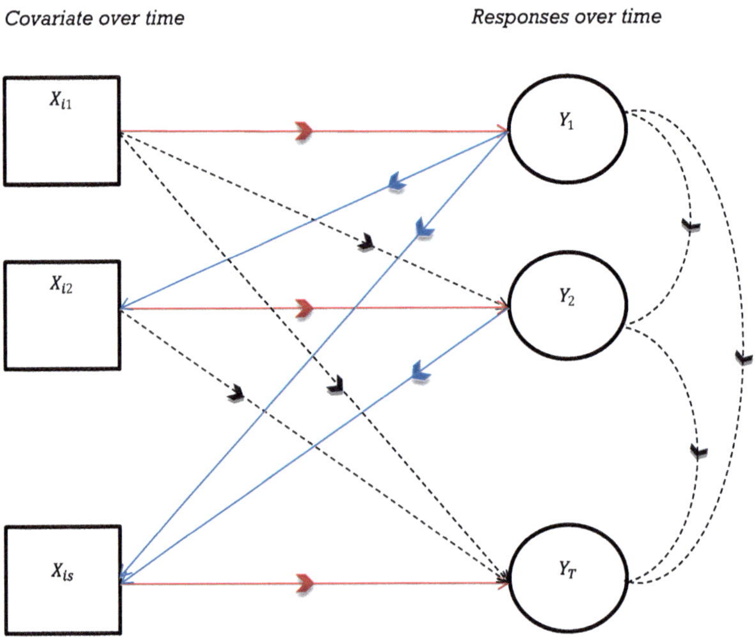

Fig. 7.1 Types of correlation structures

time period. Figure 7.1 describes two types of correlations: responses with responses and responses with covariates.

1. There is the correlation among the responses $y_1, \ldots, y_T$ as time t goes from 1 to T.
2. There is the correlation between responses at time t, Y_t and covariate values at time s, X_s:

   (a) When responses at time t impact the covariates in time t + s.
   (b) When the covariates in time t impact the responses in time t + s

These types of correlations regarding feedback from $Y_t$on to the future $X_{t+s}$and vice versa are important in obtaining the estimates of the regression coefficients when the response and covariates are not measured in the same time period. In Fig. 7.1, the arrows indicate the direction of the impact. For example, $X_{i1} \rightarrow Y_1$ denotes that X_{i1} impacts Y_1.

When analyzing longitudinal data of the kind presented in this chapter, it is essential to account both for the correlation inherent from the repeated measures of the responses and the correlation realized on account of the feedback created between the responses at a particular time and the predictors at other times. The relation between response and covariate in a linear model allows moment conditions that one may use to obtain the regression coefficients in the linear model. In particular, in cross-sectional data, the expected value of the product of the error and covariate equates to zero and is used to obtain regression coefficient estimates. However, when one encounters data collected over time and responses in different time periods are modeled with covariates in other time periods, the use of this set of moment conditions is not that straightforward. In this chapter, we present two methods (Lai & Small, 2007; Lalonde et al., 2014) that make use of all the valid moment conditions necessary with each time-dependent and time-independent covariate. The method used to determine these valid conditions is the key difference between the two methods.

Moment conditions become an issue and are not straightforward when we have a situation of feedback. The strength length of the feedback over time is not assumed to remain present at the same degree. Furthermore, we make use of continuously updating generalized method of moments (CUGMM) in obtaining these regression estimates. We fit the generalized method of moments (GMM) logistic regression model with time-dependent covariates using SAS Macro (Cai & Wilson, 2015). Since we are presented with many equations based on moment conditions from the same data, we used p-values adjusted for multiple correlated tests to determine the appropriate moment conditions for determining the regression coefficients.

7.4 Statistical Model

The use of longitudinal studies addresses, among other things, the following:

- Each unit or subject measure changes over time.
- The differences among units or subjects and their changes over time.
- The issue with longitudinal data is that they often contain repeated measurements of units or subjects at different time points.

We encounter correlated observations commonly in studies such as education, polling, healthcare, marketing, and other types of behavioral research. Among other things, the major advantage of longitudinal studies is the opportunity it affords to separate change over time within units or subjects and differences among units or subjects (cohort effects) (Diggle et al., 2002).

The challenge is when dealing with longitudinal data, the predictors or covariates can change over time besides the fact that the response variables change over time. Addressing the presence of time-dependent covariates in the analysis of longitudinal data allows the researcher to make convincing statistical inferences about the presence of any dynamic relationships and also provide more efficient estimators than if the researcher had analyzed the data as if it came from a cross-sectional dataset (Hedeker & Gibbons, 2006).

Independent observations are at the heart of the generalized linear models (GLM). As such, they are inappropriate in analyzing longitudinal data due to the clustering.

The clustering comes from the repeated measures or from the clusters or groups which results in the correlation or nonindependence. We have seen the effective use of GEE in the presence of clustering when one is fitting population-averaged logistic regression models (Liang & Zeger, 1986; Zeger & Liang, 1986; Lalonde et al., 2014).

It is common to address the analysis of longitudinal data with population-averaged models. This approach for analyzing correlated response data has received considerable attention (Zeger & Liang, 1992). Population-averaged models for longitudinal data concentrates on modeling the mean (the expectation) of a subject's response at time t as it relates to a function of the subject's covariates at time t. When the population mean parameter is the primary parameter of interest in the analysis, then marginal models are appropriate (Diggle et al., 2002) or when a function of current covariates is required to explain some property of the expectation of the response variable (Sullivan Pepe & Anderson, 1994).

In Chap. 6, we analyzed the Medicare data as it pertains to rehospitalization and repeated responses but did not give full account of the repeated measures presented on the time-dependent covariates. When there are time-dependent covariates, Hu et al. (1998) and Sullivan Pepe and Anderson (1994) have pointed out that one may not have consistent estimates when fitting GEE logistic regression models as we did in Chap. 6. This is because the covariance matrix used in the computation of the estimates is not the correct choice. While consistency is a desired property of an estimator, this may be a reason for concern unless a diagonal working covariance matrix is chosen. The need for concern is also negated if one can validate that in a given time, the marginal expectation of the response, given a particular covariate, is the same as the expectation of the response given all the covariates:

$$E\left(\left(Y_t|X_t^1\right)\right)=E\left(\left(Y_t|X_t^1,X_t^2\ldots\ldots X_t^p\right)\right)$$

where X_t^1 denotes the first covariate at time t and X_t^2 denotes the second covariate at time t and so on. In other words, if the expected value of the response given a certain covariate is equal to the case when we had that covariate as well as others were given.

In this chapter, we use the method of a moment condition equation to obtain estimates for the regression parameters in the logistic regression model. The moment condition equations are based on the expected value of the product of a covariate, and residual is zero. The residual comes from the logistic regression model based only on a model with response for rehospitalization with each of the covariates. Thus, for each parameter, there are T^2 moment conditions (given that we collected data over T times), and, hence, there are at most T^2 equations. Not all of these moments may be valid. However, all the valid moments when appropriate are combined, and we can do that through a weighted matrix based on the covariances. Such a combination of equations is not unfamiliar—it is similar to techniques done with GEE models when used for regression parameter estimates.

7.4.1 GEE Models for Time-Dependent Covariates

Even though we successfully used GEE models in Chap. 6, they are not the best choice for time-dependent covariates. In particular, Lai and Small (2007) showed that while one can combine moment conditions with time-independent covariates, this is not the case with time-dependent covariates. They showed when dealing with time-dependent covariates some of the moment conditions combined when using the generalized estimating equations with the usual arbitrary working correlation structure are not valid. More importantly, the GEE approach ignores some valid moment conditions on account of having to combine the response in one time period with the covariate of a different time period. Nevertheless, it is now an established fact that using the GEE models and treating the covariates as time-independent covariates (though it ignores some valid moments) are not as bad an approach, since the estimates provided are consistent regardless of the correlation structures for the subjects' repeated measurements. However, this is totally contingent on the selection of the correct working correlation matrix. As we saw in Chap. 6, a user-defined working correlation gives some less than satisfactory results. Recall that the GEE estimates with time-independent covariates are efficient estimates once the working correlation structure is correctly specified. The appealing fact is that the GEE estimates remain consistent and they provide the correct standard errors whether or not the working correlation structure is correctly specified.

One need not rely on selecting a working correlation, so instead of relying on GEE with its diagonal working correlation matrix, we make use of the fact that, when time-dependent covariates are present, the generalized method of moments (GMM) approach provides more efficient estimators than the GEE. We will look at a GMM approach, one based on Lalonde et al. (2014).

7.4.2 Lai and Small GMM Method

In presenting the GMM method, Lai and Small (2007), it is necessary to begin by first classifying the time-dependent covariates into one of four types. This categorization depends on the relationship existing among responses in one time period with covariates in other time periods. For convenience, we will only consider complete response data in this example, but similar procedures would apply just the same to incomplete response data.

Table 7.3 Partial data used in analysis

PNUM_R	biRadmit	NDX	NPR	LOS	DX101	Time
127	0	9	6	6	1	1
127	0	6	4	1	1	2
127	0	9	5	3	1	3
560	1	9	3	8	0	1
560	0	9	1	17	0	2
560	0	7	1	6	0	3
746	1	6	4	12	0	1
746	0	6	1	1	0	2
746	0	9	1	2	0	3
750	0	9	3	6	0	1
750	1	7	3	4	0	2
750	1	9	2	4	0	3
1117	0	9	6	5	1	1
1117	1	9	3	1	0	2
1117	0	9	6	4	1	3
1568	1	8	1	2	0	1
1568	1	9	1	4	0	2
1568	0	8	3	2	0	3
2076	1	9	5	8	1	1
2076	0	9	6	17	0	2
2076	1	9	1	6	0	3
2390	0	7	2	2	0	1
2390	0	7	2	3	0	2
2390	0	5	1	3	0	3
2413	0	9	6	17	0	1
2413	0	8	3	9	1	2
2413	0	9	2	6	0	3
3008	0	5	2	2	0	1
3008	1	6	2	3	0	2
3008	0	9	1	7	0	3

For subject *i*, example ID#560 of Table 7.3 has the response (1, 0, 0) for the three time points. Each covariate consists of a vector of values. In ID#560 NDX is (9, 9, 7) and LOS is (8, 17, 6). The data matrix consists of the covariate vector.

7.4.3 Types of Classification of Time-Dependent Covariates

Let us consider having repeated observations taken over T times on N subjects with J covariates such that $(y_{it}, x_{itj}, \ldots\ldots\ldots\ldots, x_{itJ})'$ present data for subjects i = 1, …, N; for covariates j = 1, …, J; and times t = 1, …, T; where y_{it} denotes the response for subject i at time t and x_{itj}. In the present example, T = 3, N = 1625, and J = 5 covariates (made up of NDX, LOS, DX101, and two binary variable representing time). Let us assume the marginal distribution of y_{it} conditioned on the time-dependent vector of covariates is represented by a generalized linear model. Within a particular time, there is no presence of clustering so the correlation is absent and GLM is applicable. Assume that observations y_{is} and y_{kt} are independent (different units at different times are independent). Thus, whenever $i \neq k$ (different units) but not necessarily when i = k and s ≠ t (same unit but different times). There are four conditions on which we can base the classification of the time-dependent covariates.

Condition 1: At any given time for the model $y_t = \beta_0 + \beta_1 x_t + \varepsilon_t$ the covariate x_t and the error ε_t are independent. We referred to the covariate as x_t for ease of reference, but it really refers to (all the values for a particular covariate in a certain time) x_{itj} in what follows. This is similar to the condition in regression with cross-sectional data. There are T such cases, since there are T time periods. Both the covariate and the response occur in the same time period.

Condition 2: At different times for the model $y_{t+s} = \beta_0 + \beta_1 x_t + \varepsilon_{t+s}$ the covariate x_t from an earlier period with residual from a later period is independent. Thus, the present covariates do not impact the later responses. There are $T(T - 1)/2$ such cases.

Condition 3: At different times for the model $y_t = \beta_0 + \beta_1 x_{t+s} + \varepsilon_t$ the covariates from a later period with residual from an earlier period are both independent. Thus, the responses do not impact the later covariates. There are $T(T - 1)/2$ such cases.

Collectively conditions 1, 2, and 3 are classified as type I covariates; conditions 1 and 2 collectively as type II covariates; and condition 1 as a type III covariate (Lai & Small, 2007). Covariates are classified as type IV when conditions 1 and 3 collectively are satisfied (Lalonde et al., 2014).

Lai and Small (2007) found that GMM estimates provided substantial gains in efficiency over the GEE if the covariates are type I or type II, and we suspect the same for type IV. When the covariates are type III, the estimates still remain consistent and comparable in efficiency. Thus, it is clear through omission or inclusion of moment conditions that the conclusions we make about covariates affecting our responses over time can vary. We treat the time-independent covariates as type I.

To fit GMM logistic regression models with Lai and Small's approach,

1. First identify the type of covariate, whether it is type I, type II, type III, or type IV. This differs from the method (Lalonde et al., 2014) in that the moment conditions are grouped (no test is necessarily conducted) based on the researcher's beliefs. Therefore, all the moment condition equations for that covariate are determined to be of a special type of covariate. In our example of three time periods, there are 3 × 3 = 9 equations based on type I, 3 × 2/2 = 3 equations based on type II, 3 × 2/2 = 3 equations due to type IV, and 3 equations due to type III.
2. Once we have identified the set of valid moment conditions, we can obtain the GMM estimates of the coefficients through a combination of the valid equations, thereby providing a quadratic objective function that we minimize with suitable weights.

Lalonde et al. (2014) provided a method to choose valid moment conditions when determining the effect of time-dependent covariates on binary responses. Their method does not require pre-classification of the covariates as of any particular type. While these classifications are applicable in many cases, they rely on the premise that certain correlations remain fixed and will not change even when the time between periods becomes larger. In other words, the correlation between time 1 and time 2 remains the same for time 1 and time 5.

7.4.4 Lalonde Wilson and Yin Method

However, instead of identifying covariates as types I, II, III, or IV, we could choose to treat each moment condition separately. Thus, we will fit the LWY-CUGMM (continuous updating GMM) model. To summarize, the following is how one may fit the GMM logistic regression models with the LWY-CUGMM:

1. First, for each time-dependent covariate, we identify the moment conditions associated with it. We accomplish this by examining the bivariate correlations ($\hat{\rho}_{e_t x_s}$) between the residuals and the covariate to determine the equations to use as it pertains to each covariate.
2. We take all cases of s = t as our base set of T moment conditions. They are in the same time period so the data is similar to cross sectional.
3. We then examine simultaneously the T(T − 1) moment conditions associated with s ≠ t to determine which are valid. We do that by considering at each time *t* the model:

$$\operatorname{logit}(p_t) = \beta_0 + \beta_1 x_t, \tag{7.1}$$

   where β_0 and β_1 are regression coefficients, x_t is the covariate at time t, and p_t is the probability that $y_t = 1$. Let e_t denote the residual at time t, estimating the errors at time t. Let $\hat{\rho}_{e_t x_s}$ denote the estimator for the correlation between the errors at t and the covariate at s, $\rho_{e_t x_s}$. By design we know that the correlation $\rho_{e_t x_s} = 0$ when $s = t$ but not necessarily when $s \neq t$. We posit that when $\rho_{e_t x_s} = 0$ for $s \neq t$ then the corresponding moment condition is valid.
4. This leads us to conduct a test for the correlation $\rho_{e_t x_s} = 0$ and neglect the equations for the cases when the correlations are significant. We use a method to address the multiple comparisons, thereby avoiding inflating the type I error.
5. Once we have identified the set of valid moment conditions, we obtain the GMM estimates of the coefficients through a quadratic objective function that we minimize with suitable weights.

7.5 Analysis of Data

7.5.1 Modeling Probability of Rehospitalization

Medicare is a social insurance program. It is administered by the US government. It provides health insurance coverage to people who are aged 65 and over or those who meet other special requirements. Medicare currently pays for all rehospitalizations, except those in which patients are rehospitalized within 24 h after discharge for the same condition for which they had initially been hospitalized (Jencks et al., 2009).

In analyzing these data, we chose covariates as multitude of diseases (NDX), number of procedures (NPR), length of stay (LOS), and coronary atherosclerosis (DX101). These covariates are time-dependent. The covariates associated with intercept and time indicators were treated as type I. We fit a GMM logistic regression models with time-dependent covariates to analyze these correlated data with time-dependent covariates. In analyzing these data, we first identify the appropriate and valid moment conditions associated with the time-dependent covariates and present an approach that makes use of all the valid moment conditions available with each time-dependent and time-independent covariate. In deciding which moment conditions to use, we rely on the *p*-value for the particular combination of *s* and *t* (Lalonde et al., 2014) and other techniques (Lai & Small, 2007). We engage the use of all these procedures in the SAS Macro. We fit GMM logistic regression models to the Medicare data using a SAS Macro (Cai & Wilson, 2015).

7.5.2 Modeling Probability of Rehospitalization SAS: Results

To analyze longitudinal data with binary outcomes, SAS has procedures, which utilize the statistical methods based on the generalized estimating equations (GEE) and also based on generalized linear mixed models (GLMM). We make use of a macro that fits generalized method of moments (GMM) logistic regression. This macro can appropriately take into account the correlation between covariate values (Cai & Wilson, 2015).

SAS Program

```
DATA Medicare;
Input PNUM biRadmit NDX NPR LOS DX101 Time;
Datalines;
```

127	0	9	6	6	1	1
127	0	6	4	1	1	2
127	0	9	5	3	1	3
560	1	9	3	8	0	1
560	0	9	1	17	0	2
560	0	7	1	6	0	3

```
.
;

    run;
```

Comment These are the Medicare partial data. The entire dataset is available at https://www.public.asu.edu/~jeffreyw/

```
%MVIntegration(reflib="C:\Users\Documents\Code");
```

Comment % This macro requires that the reference library (REFLIB) where an SAS catalog of the IML modules is stored is specified in the macro call. Sample code to call %MVINTEGRATION is shown:

```
%GMM(ds='C:\Users\Documents\Data',
```

Comment The second macro call to %GMM identifies the covariate types and performs generalized method of moments logistic regression.

```
        file= Medicare,
        reflib="C:\Users\Documents\Code ",
        timeVar=time,
        outVar=Radmit,
        predVar=NDX,
        predVar=NPR,
        predVar=LOS,
        predVar=DX101,
        idVar=PNUM,
        alpha=0.05);
predVar= NDX NPR LOS DX101;
```

Comment This code runs the GMM logistic regression.

```
PROC GENMOD data=Morbidity descending;
        class PNUM time(ref="1");
        model Radmit = NDX NPR LOS DX101 time / dist = bin link = logit;
        repeated subject = PNUM / within=time corr=un corrw;
 run;
```

Comment We use the SAS PROC GENMOD to model correlated data by using the REPEATED statement. This option requests generalized estimating equations to account for the presence of clustering. The GEEs are used to produce a population-averaged model, which is comparable to the GMM procedure. In this example, clustering or correlation is due to the repeated measurements on the patient (indicated by PNUM). The within patient correlation structure is specified using the CORR option. The results based on the use of PROC GENMOD is displayed.

SAS Output (Partial)

Comment The fitted GMM logistic regression model is

$$\log\left[\frac{P_1}{P_0}\right] = -0.368 + 0.065\text{NDX} - 0.031\text{NPR} + 0.034\text{LOS} - 0.114\text{DX101} - 0.388\text{T}_2 - 0.241\text{T}_3$$

The variables NDX (p = 0.0004), NPR (p = 0.0180), and LOS (p = 0.0000), as well as T_2 and T_3, are significant. GEE can be used to produce a population-averaged model, which is comparable to the GMM technique (Table 7.4).

Table 7.4 Parameter estimates/p-value based on GEE and GMM

	GEE		GMM	
Parameter	Est	P-value	Est	P-value
Intercept	−0.3675	0.0035	−0.3641	0.0034
NDX	0.0648	<0.0001	0.0543	0.0004
NPR	−0.0306	0.11	−0.0453	0.0180
LOS	0.0344	<0.0001	0.0531	0.0000
DX101	−0.1143	0.2224	0.0133	0.8878
T2	−0.3876	<0.0001	−0.4419	0.0000
T3	−0.2412	0.0005	−0.2674	0.0001

Both methods show that NDX, LOS, and time have an impact on the probability of rehospitalization. Unlike the GEE model, the GMM model find that NPR has some significant impact on the probability of rehospitalization. Unlike the GEE model, the GMM model find that NPR has some significant impact on the probability of rehospitalization.

7.6 Conclusions

When there are time-dependent covariates, we have added challenges in data analysis. This is in part mainly due to the response feedback present in the data. While the present literature has methods which allow us to address repeated measurement issues in longitudinal data, many of these methods are limited in addressing appropriately time-dependent covariates. A %GMM macro was recently developed to perform GMM logistic regression with time-dependent covariates (Cai & Wilson, 2015). This MACRO incorporates valid moment conditions through checking for significant correlation between the residuals and covariates. The approach based on GMM estimates requires one to use estimates from the GEE model and then performs an optimization with the valid moment conditions using Newton-Raphson optimization. A demonstration is performed by using the Medicare data to the fit of a GMM logistic regression model. Our results differed from our model used in Chap. 6. The standard logistic regression (Chap. 3), GEE with an unstructured working correlation matrix (Chap. 6), and GLMM (Chap. 9) produced similar results. All models failed to identify NPR as a statistically significant predictor of rehospitalization. The problem is the standard logistic regression does not appropriately handle the repeated observations, nor does it address the time-dependent covariates, since many of the valid moment conditions are left out. The GEE method is not assured to have consistent estimators when using time-dependent covariates, as it models the correlation as a nuisance parameter in the random component, and GLMM similarly is unable to produce appropriate estimates.

Most researchers are aware of the consequences when analyzing repeated binary measures data; the correlations present on account of the repeated measures in the responses are addressed. However, until recent times, most researchers have ignored the dependency also present in the covariates that changes over time due to factors other than natural growth. In general, the modeling of repeated measures data must address the two sets of correlation inherent: one due to the responses and the other due to the covariates. The generalized method of moments is an alternative choice over GEE with an independent working correlation matrix. One can easily fit GMM logistic regression models with SAS Macro but may choose to use PROC IML. The GMM approach is appropriate for marginal models for time-dependent covariates, both for binary and nonbinary responses. Interestingly, Lalonde et al. (2014) showed that incorrectly specifying the type of covariate may result in significant changes in the standard errors and thereby lead to erroneous conclusions. Most researchers realize that in the analysis of repeated binary measures data, the correlations present on account of the repeated measures in the responses are addressed.

7.7 Related Examples

Data collected by the International Food Policy Research Institute in the Bukidnon Province in the Philippines were analyzed by Lai and Small (2007) and later Lalonde et al. (2014). They analyzed data consisting of body mass index (BMI) and morbidity measured for 370 children at 3 separate time points, separated by 4-month intervals. The study purpose was to predict morbidity for children over time based on various factors. There is a total of 1110 observations, with 3 different BMI measurements for each of the 370 children. For children (labeled by childID), the visit number (time) and the body mass index (BMI) are taken and recorded. For each of the three visits, the child was sick (sick = 1) or healthy (sick = 0) at the time of measurement. There is additional information collected in the study, pertaining prediction of morbidity based on the visit number and the child's BMI. These data can be analyzed based on the models presented in this chapter.

References

Cai, K., & Wilson, J. R. (2015). *How to use SAS for GMM logistic regression models for longitudinal data with time-dependent covariates* (SUGI Paper 3252-2015).

Cohen, J., Cohen, P., West, S. G., & Aiken, L. S. (2003). *Applied multiple regression/correlation analysis for the behavioral sciences* (3rd ed.). Erlbaum.

Diggle, P., Heagerty, P., Liang, K., & Zeger, S. (2002). *Analysis of longitudinal data* (p. 485). Oxford University Press.

Hansen, L. P. (1982). Large sample properties of generalized method of moments estimators. *Econometrica, 50*(4), 1029–1054.

Hansen, L. P., Heaton, J., & Yaron, A. (1996). Finite-sample properties of some alternative GMM estimators. *Journal of Business and Economic Statistics, 14*(3), 262–280.

Hays, W. L. (1994). *Statistics* (5th ed.). Harcourt Brace College Publishers.

Hedeker, D., & Gibbons, R. D. (2006). *Longitudinal data analysis*. Wiley-Interscience.

Hu, F. B., Goldberg, J., Hedeker, D., Flay, B. R., & Pentz, M. A. (1998). Comparison of population-averaged and subject-specific approaches for analyzing repeated binary outcomes. *American Journal of Epidemiology, 147*(7), 694–703.

Jencks, S. F., Williams, M. V., & Coleman, E. A. (2009). Rehospitalizations among patients in the Medicare fee-for-service program. *New England Journal of Medicine, 360*(14), 1418–1428.

Lai, T. L., & Small, D. (2007). Marginal regression analysis of longitudinal data with time-dependent covariates: A generalized method-of-moments approach. *Journal of the Royal Statistical Society: Series B (Statistical Methodology), 69*(1), 79–99.

Lalonde, T., Nguyen, A. Q., Yin, J., Irimata, K., & Wilson, J. R. (2014). Modeling correlated binary outcomes with time-dependent covariates. *Journal of Data Science, 11*(4), 715–738.

Lalonde, T., Wilson, J. R., & Yin, J. (2014, November). GMM logistic regression models for longitudinal data with time-dependent covariates and extended classifications. *Statistics in Medicine, 33*(27), 4756–4769.

Liang, K. Y., & Zeger, S. L. (1986). Longitudinal data analysis using generalized linear models. *Biometrika, 73*(1), 13–22.
Maxwell, S. E., & Delaney, H. D. (2000). *Designing experiments and analyzing data.* Erlbaum.
Sullivan Pepe, M., & Anderson, G. L. (1994). A cautionary note on inference for marginal regression models with longitudinal data and general correlated response data. *Communications in Statistics-Simulation and Computation, 23*(4), 939–951.
Zeger, S. L., & Liang, K. Y. (1986). Longitudinal data analysis for discrete and continuous outcomes. *Biometrics, 42*(1), 121–130.
Zeger, S. L., & Liang, K. Y. (1992). An overview of methods for the analysis of longitudinal data. *Statistics in Medicine, 11*(14–15), 1825–1839.

Chapter 8
Exact Logistic Regression Model

8.1 Motivating Example

A recent study of the effect of phensic aspirin on migraine involved 16 patients. Eight of the 16 patients received the phensic aspirin, and the others received a placebo. The patients were observed for a period of 4 h, and whether or not they got relief for a certain time was compared with the non-phensic pill. The data are summarized in Table 8.1.

Later, we learned that the patients were not randomly assigned but rather were clustered in groups of four where some groups were under a physician's care and some self-monitored. This study consisted of a small sample size, and it appears that the observations are not necessarily independent, but clustered. As such we present the exact logistic regression. This technique is appropriate because the outcome variable is binary, the sample size is small, and some cells are empty. The standard logistic regression relies on asymptotic theory, so small sample size and the presence of cells with no subjects make regular logistic regression not advisable, and it might not even be estimable.

The increase in computer capacity makes the use of exact methods to analyze data increasingly popular in healthcare, banking, and other industries. This is a result of the fact that the traditional methods (which are based on asymptotic theory) for analyzing small, skewed, or sparse datasets are not always reliable. In fact, the asymptotic methods are inadequate when sample sizes are small or when the data are sparse or skewed. In such cases exact conditional inference is necessary and applicable (Derr, 2000). We also examine the analysis of small sample size data, when the sample data were collected based on correlated observations. In addition, one may also wonder how we analyze small sample data, if the sample data were based on a one-stage clustering, two-stage clustering, or higher levels of clustering. We address exact methods for both small sample with independent observations and also with correlated observations in this chapter.

J. R. Wilson et al., *Modeling Binary Correlated Responses*, ICSA Book Series in Statistics, https://doi.org/10.1007/978-3-031-62427-8_8

Table 8.1 Summary data for phensic aspirin study

	Phensic aspirin	Non-phensic aspirin
Relief	3	1
No relief	5	7

The exact methods of inferences are based on enumerating the exact distributions of certain statistics to estimate the parameters of interest in a logistic regression model, conditional on the remaining parameters. While asymptotic theory allows us to fit certain statistical models to large datasets, it is not applicable to small or sparse datasets. However, when confronted with small datasets in a multivariable setting, the inclination by some non-statisticians is to either analyze two variables at a time or ignore the warnings and proceed.

8.2 Definition and Notation

Asymptotic theory or as some refer to as large sample theory is a method referring to the behavior or properties of estimators and the statistical test that they gave rise to. Asymptotic theory tells how these estimators behave when the sample size (for appropriate subpopulation) is sufficiently large.

Exact logistic regression is a useful tool to model binary outcome in which the logit or log odds of the outcome are modeled as a linear combination of the predictor variables. The exact model is used when the sample sizes are too small for the standard logistic regression (recall the standard logistic regression model relies on the maximum likelihood-based estimation) and/or when some of the cells' frequencies are zero. The exact method is void of asymptotic theory. For example, the Pearson's chi-square test is not exact because the distribution of the test statistic is satisfied only asymptotically.

Parametric tests are exact tests when the parametric assumptions are fully met. It has become the norm to use *exact* (significance) *test* for those tests that do not rest on parametric assumptions. So we adopt the school of thought that when the result of a statistical analysis is said to be an "exact test" or an "exact p-value" and that the test is defined without parametric assumptions and evaluated without using approximate algorithms (Siegel, 1957).

Fisher's exact test is exact because the sampling distribution, conditional on the marginal, is known exactly.

Sufficient statistic is a simple function of the data, for example, the sum of all the data points. It is sufficient such that "no other statistic which can be calculated from the same sample provides any additional information pertaining to the value of the parameter." For a given unknown parameter, a sufficient statistic is a function whose value contains all the information needed to compute any estimate of the parameter.

Ancillary statistics A_s, is called an ancillary statistic for parameter θ means the distribution of A_s does not depend on θ.

Clustered data occur frequently in statistical practice. In some areas of application, clustered data are the rule rather than the exception. An example is in ophthalmology. In such a setting, standard logistic regression models are invalid, due to the lack of independence among responses for individual sample points within a cluster, the left and right eye.

Exact methods date back to the Fisher's exact test for 2 × 2 tables and the multi hypergeometric version for larger dimensions. Corcoran et al. (2001) and Troxler et al. (2011) presented exact methods to analyze correlated data.

The *penalized log likelihood* can be seen as a method for measuring the conflict between smoothness and goodness-of-fit to the data. *Penalized maximum likelihood* estimation (PMLE) is "a more rigorous method because adjustment for over fitting is directly built into the model development, instead of relying on shrinkage afterward." Penalized Maximum Likelihood Estimation to predict binary outcomes: Moons, K. G., Donders, A. R., Steyerberg, E. W., & Harrell, F. E. (2004). *Journal of Clinical Epidemiology*, *57*(12), 1262–1270.

8.3 Exploratory Analysis

8.3.1 Artificial Data for Clustering

We have a somewhat artificial set of data based on some real (but without permission to use fully publicly) experiments conducted by the statistics research group at Arizona State University, W.P. Carey School of Business. The data are void of its real names to protect the sensitivity and the lack of permission to use with identifiers. However, these data have a known nested correlation structure. The data with its generic names are given in Table 8.2. In Table 8.2, we have the information for one-stage clustered data where n_i denotes the number of units in cluster i, z_i is the total number of events in cluster i, and x_i is the covariate value for cluster i. We want to fit a logistic regression model logit $[p_{ij}] = \beta_0 + \beta_1 x_i$, where $p_{ij} = 1$ is the probability of a positive response for outcome j in cluster i.

8.3.2 Standard Logistic Regression

If we were to ignore the clustering and only concentrate on the size of the data, we can present the data as in the last two columns of Table 8.2. Then the test for significance of the covariate X is all nonsignificant ($p > 0.2189$). The fitted standard

Table 8.2 Generic data for one-stage cluster

Cluster	Number n_i	Count z_i	x_i	Response probability	Covariate
1	4	2	2	0.50	2
2	2	0	4	0.00	4
3	6	2	3	0.33	3

logistic regression model is logit (P_i) = 2.61 − 1.21X and the odds ratio is [0.037, 2.403]. The covariate has no significant impact on the response. The fit of logistic regression models to independent binary data has relied heavily on asymptotic theory (see Chap. 3) and to a lesser extent on exact distributions in the case of small samples.

Sparse and Skewed Correlated Binary Data

The fit of logistic regression models to correlated binary data based on an exact distribution is not as common. Some attention has been given to one-stage clustered data as opposed to higher dimensions as there is less complexity. When statistical inferences for studies involve large sample approximations, the fit of logistic regression models is performed through the unconditional likelihood function. However, when the data are sparse, exact methods of estimation, based on sufficient statistics, are generally preferred. The large sample theory estimates have been shown to be unreliable when data are sparse or skewed or display complete separation, or there are many covariates relative to the number of observations (Troxler et al., 2011).

Cox (1970) suggested computing the conditional distribution of the sufficient statistics for the parameters of interest over all possible outcomes that lead to the observed values of the ancillary statistics. This method, at times, may involve a number of parameters, having exponential growth relative to the sample size, and as such may prove time consuming. Derr (2000) and Mehta and Patel (1995) have given a complete description of the theoretical aspects of exact logistic regression model with a discussion of its implementation. Mehta and Patel (1995) pointed out the major differences between the results based on the exact method as compared to those based on maximum likelihood estimation.

8.3.3 *Two-Stage Clustered Data*

In Table 8.3, we have a two-stage clustered data, where "cluster" labels the first-stage clusters, n_{ij} denotes the number of observations in each cluster, z_{ij} is the number of positive responses in each cluster, and the predictor is x_{ij}. Our interest is fitting an exact logistic regression model to such data. Mehta and Patel (1995) examined the analysis of binary data using the logistic model with independent observations, but the issues due to correlated observations have received less attention. Connolly and Liang (1988), among others, have proposed methods of performing large sample logistic estimation when the observations are correlated, but exact methods for correlated data have not become the focal point until recent times. In practice, the use of the standard logistic model to analyze independent binary data depends for the most part on asymptotic theory in large samples, and we usually reserve the exact distributions for small samples. However, the use of logistic models for correlated data based on exact analysis is not as common. In fact, the common practice when confronted with two-stage and higher level is usually to apply the data as

Table 8.3 Generic data for two-stage cluster

Cluster	Number n_{ij}	Count z_{ij}	x_{ij}
1	4	2	2
1	2	0	4
1	6	2	3
2	5	0	0
2	5	0	1
3	3	1	7
3	7	6	6
3	4	2	7
3	2	1	5

obtained from one-stage clustering. In this chapter, we use an exact method of analysis to address hypothesis testing (estimation is not addressed) for data with second-stage and probably higher levels of clustering. We allow correlation among observations within the one-stage model. We present the models with a single covariate. We examine cases when the covariates differ within clusters in a two-stage binomial model (Troxler et al., 2011). Computations using the C++ programming are given in http://www.public.asu.edu/~jeffreyw.

8.4 Statistical Models

8.4.1 Independent Observations

When analyzing data with independent observations, Cox (1970) proposed a method for dealing with sparse data. This method is based on treating some of the regression parameters of interest and the other parameters as nuisance parameters. This approach relies in part on the fact that the logistic regression model has its random component belonging to the exponential family which can be used to determine sufficient statistics for the parameters of interest and ancillary statistics sufficient for the nuisance parameters. We used the method as available in SAS with EXACT option to analyze. We direct the reader interested in the development of this method and procedure to see SAS manual PROC FREQ Chap. 28. We also use R to fit the exact logistic regression.

8.4.2 One-Stage Cluster Model

An exact method for clustered data by relying on the conditioning arguments similar to that which was used with exponential family models for samples of independent observations was proposed (Troxler et al., 2011). Consider the data for the one-stage cluster in Table 8.4 (a revision of Table 8.2), and fit the logistic regression

Table 8.4 Generic data for one-stage cluster

Cluster	Number n_i	Count z_i			x_i	
1	4	2	2	2(4–2)	2	2(2)
2	2	0	0	0(2–0)	4	0(4)
3	6	2	2	2(6–2)	3	2(3)
		$\sum_j z_j = 4$	$s_1 = 4$	$s_2 = 12$		t = 10

model logit $[p_i] = \alpha + \beta x_i$. To fit such model with exact analysis, we demonstrate using data from Table 8.2 but computed in Table 8.4.

There are three clusters. We have the sample size n_i for each cluster and the number of events z_i in each cluster. Let the reference set $\Gamma(s_1, s_2)$ contain all possible outcomes of z_i that would have resulted in the observed values for s_1, and s_2. So based on Table 8.4, $s_1 = 2 + 0 + 2 = 4$ and $s_2 = 2(2) + 0(2) + 2(4) = 12$ and $t = 2(2) + 0(4) + 2(3) = 10$. The set $\Gamma(s_1, s_2)$ consists of all cases where $\sum_j z_j = 4$ such that $s_1 = 4$ and $s_2 = 12$. Thus, the set $\Gamma(s_1, s_2)$ is given in Table 8.5.

Thus, a conditional distribution argument can be used to test H_o the null hypothesis against H_a the alternative hypothesis, i.e., $H_o: \beta = 0$ against H_a: $\beta > 0$. Under H_o, the conditional distribution of Z = z reduces to

$$\Pr\left(Z_i = z_i \middle| x_i; s_1, s_2\right) = \frac{\prod_{i=1}^{N} \binom{n_i}{z_i}}{\sum_{z^* \in \Gamma(s_1, s_2)} \prod_{i=1}^{N} \binom{n_i}{z_i^*}} \tag{8.1}$$

$$\Pr\left(Z_i = 4 \middle| x_i; 4, 12\right) = \frac{\binom{2}{2}\binom{4}{0}\binom{3}{2}}{\binom{2}{2}\binom{4}{0}\binom{3}{2} + \binom{2}{1}\binom{4}{0}\binom{3}{3} + \binom{2}{1}\binom{4}{1}\binom{3}{2}}$$

$$= \frac{3}{3 + 2 + 24} = 0.103448, \text{with } t = 10.$$

Since the likelihood ratio is decreasing in t, a one-sided p-value for this test is

$$\Pr\left(t > t_{obs} \middle| H_0, x, s\right) = \sum_{z^* \in \Gamma(s_1, s_2): t(z^*) \geq t} \left[\frac{\prod_{i=1}^{N} \binom{n_i}{z_i}}{\sum_{z^* \in \Gamma(s_1, s_2)} \prod_{i=1}^{N} \binom{n_i}{z_i^*}} \right]$$

$$= 0.069(\text{t} = 11) + 0.827(\text{t} = 12) = 0.896$$

Table 8.5 Generic data for one-stage cluster

	Cluster 1	Cluster 2	Cluster 3	$n_1 - z_1$	$n_2 - z_2$	$n_3 - z_3$	s_1	s_2	t
	0	0	4	4	2	2	4	8	12
	0	1	3	4	1	3	4	10	13
	0	2	2	4	0	4	4	8	14
	1	2	1	3	0	5	4	8	13
$\Gamma(s_1, s_2)$	**1**	**1**	**2**	**3**	**1**	**4**	**4**	**12**	12
$\Gamma(s_1, s_2)$	**1**	**0**	**3**	**3**	**2**	**3**	**4**	**12**	11
$\Gamma(s_1, s_2)$	**2**	**0**	**2**	**2**	**2**	**4**	**4**	**12**	10
	3	0	1	1	2	5	4	8	9
	3	1	0	1	1	6	4	4	10
	4	0	0	0	2	6	4	0	8

We reject H_0 if the p-value is less than our significance level α. In http://www.public.asu.edu/~jeffreyw, we provide the C^{++} program to compute the p-values.

8.4.3 Two-Stage Cluster Exact Logistic Regression Model

Similarly, Troxler et al. (2011) also presented the case of two stages of clustering, where the design consists of second-stage clusters nested within the first-stage clusters. We demonstrate this fit with the data in Table 8.3 and reproduce their results.

Let Y_{ijk} be the kth observation from the jth secondary cluster contained in the ith primary cluster ($i = 1, 2 \ldots n; j = 1, 2, \ldots, n_i; k = 1, 2, \ldots, n_{ij}$). Let the value of the covariate for all observations in the ijth secondary cluster be x_{ij}. Let $Z_{ij} = \sum_{k=1}^{n_{ij}} Y_{ijk}$, with $s_1 = \sum_{i=1}^{n}\sum_{j=1}^{n_i} z_{ij}$, with $s_2 = \sum_{i=1}^{n}\sum_{j=1}^{n_i} z_{ij}\left(n_{ij} - z_{ij}\right)$ and $s_3 = \sum_{i=1}^{n}\left[\sum_{j=1}^{n_i} z_{ij}\left[\sum_{j=1}^{n_i}\left(n_{ij} - z_{ij}\right)\right]\right]$ with $t = \left[\sum_{j=1}^{n_i} x_{ij} z_{ij}\right]$. Let $\Gamma(s_1, s_2, s_3)$ contain all possible outcomes of Z_i that would have resulted in the observed values for s_1, s_2 and s_3. To address statistical tests or inferences about β in $logit\,[p_i] = \alpha + \beta x_i$ we focus on the conditional distribution of the sufficient statistic t, given the observed values of the sufficient statistics s_1, s_2, and s_3. Then the conditional distribution of $Z_i = z_i$ reduces to

$$\Pr\left(Z_i = z_i \middle| x; s_1, s_2, s_3\right) = \frac{\prod_{i=1}^{K}\prod_{i=1}^{I}\prod_{j=1}^{J_i}\binom{n_{ij}}{z_{ij}}}{\sum_{z^* \in \Gamma(s_1, s_2, s_3)}\prod_{i=1}^{I}\prod_{j=1}^{J_i}\binom{n_{ij}}{z_{ij}}} \tag{8.2}$$

Thus, the likelihood ratio for $\beta = 0$ versus $\beta > 0$ is decreasing in t, so a one-sided p-value for this test is

$$\Pr\left(t > t_{obs} | H_0, x, s\right) = \sum_{z^* \in \Gamma(s_1, s_2, s_3): t(z^*) \geq t_{obs}} \left[\frac{\prod_{i=1}^{K} \prod_{i=1}^{I} \prod_{j=1}^{J_i} \binom{n_{ij}}{z_{ij}}}{\sum_{z^* \in \Gamma(s_1, s_2, s_3)} \prod_{i=1}^{I} \prod_{j=1}^{J_i} \binom{n_{ij}}{z_{ij}}} \right]$$

Thus, we reject H_0 if the p-value is less than our significance level α or, equivalently, if $t_{obs} > t_\alpha$, where t_α is the smallest value of t for which Pr $(t > t_{obs} | H_0, \boldsymbol{x}, \boldsymbol{s}) \leq \alpha$. Exact logistic regression models with correlated data requires lots of memory in computing, and as such it is relatively easy to exceed the memory capacity of a given computer (Troxler et al., 2011). We run these models with our C^{++} program as given in http://www.public.asu.edu/~jeffreyw.

8.5 Analysis of Data

We used exact logistic regression models for nested binary data to fit the data in Tables 8.2 and 8.3 (Troxler et al., 2011). This technique is appropriate because the outcome variable is binary, the sample size is small, and data are sparse. As such, standard logistic regression is not reliable due to the small sample size and the presence of cells with no values. In fact, the cell probabilities might not even be estimable. We fit a logistic regression model logit(p) = α + βx, where p is the probability of a single positive response for the data in Table 8.3. We use SAS and R.

Exact logistic regression is used to model binary outcome variables in which the log odds of the outcome is modeled as a linear combination of the predictor variables. It is used when the sample size is too small for a regular logistic regression (which uses the standard maximum likelihood-based estimator) and/or when some of the cells formed by the outcome and categorical predictor variable have no observations. The estimates given by exact logistic regression do not depend on asymptotic results. Our data suggest that response is zero or one. We have the group it belongs to and the covariate X. Table 8.6 consists of the data in grouped form, while Table 8.7 has the data in ungrouped form.

We are interested in how does the covariate X impact the response, but taking the group into account. The outcome variable is binary (0/1): 0 or 1. The predictor variable of interest is X, and the group can be seen as a nuisance variable. We need to use a model that handles binary outcome variables correctly when the data are sparse. Also, because the number of individuals in a group is small, we will need a method that can perform the estimation with a small sample size.

Table 8.6 Grouped data for response with covariate X

Group	Total	#Events	X
1	4	2	2
1	2	0	4
1	6	2	3
2	5	0	0
2	5	0	1
3	3	1	7
3	7	6	6
3	4	2	7
3	2	1	5

8.5.1 Exact Logistic Regression for Independent Observations

The exact conditional logistic regression model was fitted using the LOGISTIC procedure in SAS. It provides two tests for the null hypothesis that the parameters are zero: the exact probability test and the exact conditional score test used. It gives a test statistic, an exact *p*-value, and a mid *p*-value that adjusts for the discreteness of the distribution. In addition, it gives individual hypothesis tests for the parameter of each continuous effect and joint tests for the parameters of classification variable (Jones & Huddleston, 2009). Consider fitting logit $[p_i] = \alpha + \beta x_i$. The data have sample size which is small.

8.5.2 Exact Logistic Regression for One-Stage Clustered Data

Using SAS, we have

SAS Program

```
DATA chap8;
INPUT GROUP N COUNT X;
*Data from Table 8.3 for two-stage clustered;
DATALINES;
```

1	4	2	2
1	2	0	4
1	6	2	3
2	5	0	0
2	5	0	1
3	3	1	7
3	7	6	6
3	4	2	7
3	2	1	5

Table 8.7 Ungrouped data for response with covariate X

Group	Event	x
1	1	2
1	1	2
1	0	2
1	0	2
1	0	4
1	0	4
1	1	3
1	1	3
1	0	3
1	0	3
1	0	3
1	0	3
2	0	0
2	0	0
2	0	0
2	0	0
2	0	0
2	0	1
2	0	1
2	0	1
2	0	1
2	0	1
3	1	7
3	0	7
3	0	7
3	1	6
3	1	6
3	1	6
3	1	6
3	1	6
3	1	6
3	0	6
3	1	7
3	1	7
3	0	7
3	0	7
3	1	5
3	0	5

```
;
PROC LOGISTIC DATA = chap8 DESC;
MODEL COUNT/N= X/ firth clodds=pl;
  ods output cloddspl=firth;
EXACT X/ ESTIMATE = BOTH; RUN;
```

Comment We conducted the exact logistic analysis using PROC LOGISTIC with the EXACT statement. We included the option estimate = BOTH on the EXACT statement. That allowed us to obtain both the point estimates and the odds ratios in the output.

SAS Output

The LOGISTIC procedure	
Model information	
Dataset	WORK.CHAP8
Response variable (events)	COUNT
Response variable (trials)	N
Model	Binary logit
Optimization technique	Fisher's scoring
Likelihood penalty	Firth's bias correction
Number of observations read	9
Number of observations used	9
Sum of frequencies read	38
Sum of frequencies used	38

Comment There are nine rows in the table. There are 38 responses. These results are not related to asymptotic or to exact methods.

Response profile		
Ordered value	Binary outcome	Total frequency
1	Event	14
2	Nonevent	24

Comment There are 14 of the 38 who responded as an event, "1." This is a small dataset.

Intercept only model convergence status			
Convergence criterion (GCONV = 1E-8) satisfied			
Model convergence status			
Convergence criterion (GCONV = 1E-8) satisfied			
Model fit statistics			
Criterion	Intercept only	Intercept and covariates	
		Log likelihood	Full log likelihood
AIC	45.823	40.301	20.243
SC	47.460	43.577	23.518
−2 Log L	43.823	36.301	16.243

Comment These tests give the value with and without the covariates. The difference provides a test of the significance of the simultaneous effect of the covariates.

Testing global null hypothesis: Beta = 0			
Test	Chi-square	DF	Pr > ChiSq
Likelihood ratio	7.5213	1	0.0061
Score	7.5246	1	0.0061
Wald	5.9699	1	0.0146

Comment Predictor X is significant (p = 0.0146; p = 0.0061) in the model. These p-values were obtained on the large sample theory based on independent observations.

Analysis of penalized maximum likelihood estimates					
Parameter	DF	Estimate	Std. error	Wald chi-square	Pr > ChiSq
Intercept	1	−2.0854	0.7838	7.0796	0.0078
X	1	0.3935	0.1610	5.9699	0.0146

Comment The model logit ($P_{response=1}$) = −2.0854 + 0.3935 X is the fitted logistic regression model with a significant covariate. The coefficient estimates are based on the penalized maximum likelihood estimates. This makes adjustment for the challenge between goodness-of-fit and smoothness. The *likelihood ratio* and the *score test* showed that the covariate is significant.

Odds ratio estimates and profile-likelihood confidence intervals				
Effect	Unit	Estimate	95% confidence limits	
X	1.0000	1.482	1.112	2.089

Comment Through the confidence intervals based on the profile-likelihood, the odds ratio lies between 1.112 and 2.089. But these are based on a distribution of the responses. This confidence interval is plotted in the following graph. These results assume that the usual assumptions are satisfied.

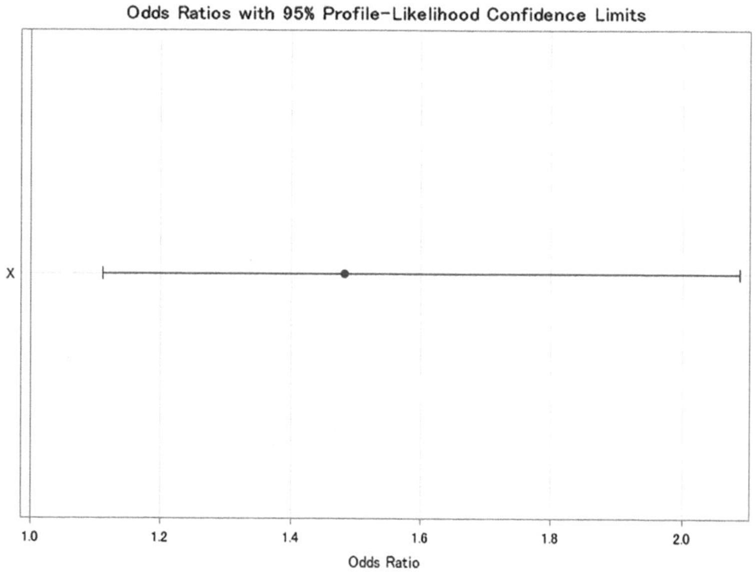

Comment This confidence interval is based on the profile-likelihood method and not on the exact methods.

The Logistic Procedure

Exact conditional analysis				
Exact conditional tests				
Effect	Test	Statistic	p-value	
			Exact	Mid
X	Score	7.3876	0.0067	0.0061
	Probability	0.00124	0.0067	0.0061

Comment For each parameter estimate, the procedure displays either the exact maximum conditional likelihood estimates or the median unbiased estimate. In addition, the exponential of the estimate, the one- or two-sided confidence limits, and a one- or two-sided p-value for testing that the parameter is equal to zero are displayed.

Exact parameter estimates					
Parameter	Estimate	Standard error	95% confidence limits		Two-sided p-value
X	0.4149	0.1634	0.1028	0.7779	0.0069

Comment The hypothesis tests can be generated for each individual effect in an EXACT statement or for all effects simultaneously. However, parameter estimates are computed for each effect individually. There are two tests for the null hypothesis that the parameters for the effects specified in the EXACT statement are zero: the exact probability test and the exact conditional score test. For each test used, the "conditional exact tests" table displays the following:—a test statistic—an exact p-value, which is the probability of obtaining a more extreme statistic than the observed value, assuming the null hypothesis—a mid p-value, which adjusts for the discreteness of the distribution parameter estimates and odds ratios for each effect in the EXACT statement conditional on the values of all the other parameters in the model. Predictor X is significant (p = 0.0069). This is the exact method based on independent observations.

Exact odds ratios				
Parameter	Estimate	95% confidence limits		Two-sided p-value
X	1.514	1.108	2.177	0.0069

Comment The hypothesis tests can be generated for each individual effect in an EXACT statement or for all effects simultaneously. The intercept is not included in the output because its sufficient statistic was conditioned out when creating the joint distribution of the predictor. The predictor is significant in the model (p = 0.0069). The odds ratio ranged from [1.108, 2.177].

```
PROC LOGISTIC DATA = chap8 DESC;
MODEL COUNT/N= X/ firth clodds=pl;
   ods output cloddspl=firth;
EXACT X/ ESTIMATE = BOTH;
output out = ch8_predicted pred = predicted;
RUN;
```

Group	N	Count	X	Predicted
1	4	2	2	0.214419
1	2	0	4	0.374826
1	6	2	3	0.288018
2	5	0	0	0.110523
2	5	0	1	0.155519
3	3	1	7	0.661238
3	7	6	6	0.568407
3	4	2	7	0.661238
3	2	1	5	0.470507

The exact logistic regression is appropriate because the outcome variable is binary, the sample size is small, and some cells are empty. The standard logistic regression will not perform well due to the small sample size and the presence of cells with no units, and it might not even be estimable. We fitted the data in Table 8.6 using exact logistic regression analysis using R with elrm package.

8.5.3 Exact Logistic Regression for Independent Observations with R Programming

R Program

```
> elrm.out = elrm(Count/N ~ X, interest = ~ X, iter = 22000,
burnIn = 2000, dataset = ch8)
> summary(elrm.out)
Call:
[[1]] elrm(formula = Count/N ~ X, interest = ~X, iter = 22000,
dataset = ch8, burnIn = 2000)
```

Comment elrm implements a modification proposed by Forster et al. (2003) to approximate exact conditional inference for logistic regression models. The modifications can handle larger datasets. Exact conditional inference is based on the distribution of the sufficient statistics for the parameters of interest given the sufficient statistics for the remaining nuisance parameters. Using model formula notation, users specify a logistic model and model terms of interest for exact inference (ELRM package in R).

```
Results:
        estimate      p-value      p-value_se      mc_size
X       0.41503       0.0036       0.00084         20000
            95% Confidence Intervals for Parameters
                  lower                  upper
X               0.1032715              0.8773408
```

8.5.4 Exact Logistic Regression for One-Stage Clustered Data with R Program

Data in Table 8.2 were obtained from a one-stage cluster.

R Program
This was fitted using an R program (http://www.public.asu.edu/~jeffreyw) that allows an exhaustive search through all possible outcomes to compute the conditional distribution.

R Output
We first fit the model of [1], *logit* $[p_i] = \alpha + \beta x_i$ using the probability mass function 8.1 and 8.2, ignoring the first-stage clustering of *group*. The p-value for the one-sided parameter test $H_0 : \beta = 0$ *vs* $H_a : \beta > 0$ is $p_1 = 0.033$. The model described in Sect. 8.4 was also fitted using probability mass function 10, where the *group* level of correlation is accounted for in the model. The p-value for the one-sided parameter test is now $p_2 = 0.095$.

Comment The test statistic for the model with only first-stage clustering is clearly inflated by ignoring the additional level of clustering built into the data. The R program was unable to complete this calculation.

8.5.5 *Exact Logistic Regression for One-Stage Clustered Data with C++ Program*

C++ Program
The data were analyzed using a C++ program (http://www.public.asu.edu/~jeffreyw) (reproduced here for ease of reference) which can handle larger datasets than the R program. In addition to being faster and more efficient with memory, the C++ program uses feasibility checks, to avoid computing the entire distribution. These feasibility checks allow the use of reasonably large datasets when the total number of successes remains small.

C++ Output
The data in Table 8.3 were analyzed similarly to the data in Table 8.2. The model described was fitted using probability mass function, where the group level of correlation is accounted for in the model. The C++ program computed the one-sided p-value of 0.0085 for the test of $H_o : \beta = 0$ against $H_a : \beta > 0$ in *logit* $[p_i] = \alpha + \beta x_i$. The R program was unable to complete this calculation.

Comment Exact logistic regression is a very memory intensive procedure, and it is relatively easy to exceed the memory capacity of a given computer. Exact logistic regression is an alternative to conditional logistic regression if you have stratification, since both conditioned on the number of positive outcomes within each stratum. The estimates from these two analyses will be different because conditional logit conditions only on the intercept term, while exact logistic regression conditions on the sufficient statistics of the other regression parameters as well as the intercept term (www.ats.ucla.edu/stat/sas/dae/exlogit.htm).

8.5.6 *Exact Logistic Regression for Two-Stage Clustered Data with C++ Program*

C++ Program
The data were analyzed using a C++ program (http://www.public.asu.edu/~jeffreyw) (and reproduced here for ease of reference) which can handle larger datasets than

the R program. In addition, to being faster and more efficient with memory, the C++ program uses feasibility checks, to avoid computing the entire distribution. These feasibility checks allow the use of reasonably large datasets when the total number of successes remains small.

C++ Output
The data in Table 8.7 were analyzed similarly to the data in Table 8.6. The model described was fitted using probability mass function (Sect. 8.4), where the group level of correlation is accounted for in the model. The C++ program computed the one-sided p-value of 0.0085 for the test of $H_0\colon\beta = 0$ *vs* $H_a\colon\beta > 0$. For cases in which the dataset may be very small, as in Table 8.2, an exhaustive program will suffice. But for a situation as in Table 8.3, where the probability of a success is very low, the more efficient program is necessary. In fact, even with reasonably large sample sizes, the asymptotic theory will not apply well. In this case, for Table 8.7, the asymptotic generalized moment conditions approach fails to produce positive definite covariance structures for parameter estimates, but our exact method is able to perform a one-sided hypothesis test.

8.6 Conclusions

The use of large sample theory for fitting logistic models is well documented both for correlated and for uncorrelated observations. However, the use of exact analysis is not as well known. This chapter presented exact models for correlated sparse data through different levels of clustering. We reviewed a one-sided test, $H_0\colon\beta = 0$ *vs* $H_a\colon\beta > 0$. To conduct the test $H_0\colon\beta = 0$ *vs* $H_a\colon\beta < 0$, in $logit\,[p_i] = \alpha + \beta x_i$ we could either perform the given test using $Y_{ij}^{'} = 1 - Y_{ij}$, or we could equivalently use a p-value obtained by summing over $t < t_{obs}$ instead of $t > t_{obs}$. However, to conduct a two-sided test of $H_0\colon\beta = 0$ *vs* $H_a\colon\beta \neq 0$ given that the conditional distribution of t is not symmetric, we should find $t_{\alpha/2}$ and $t_{1-\alpha/2}$where, for $0 < p < 1$, t_p is the smallest value of t' satisfying $Pr\,(t < t'\colon H_0, x, s) \geq p$. We reject the null hypothesis if the observed value of t, t_{obs} is either greater than $t_{1-\alpha/2}$ or less than $t_{\alpha/2}$.

8.7 Related Examples

Consider this hypothetical situation. Suppose that we are interested in the factors that influence whether or not an executive is admitted into the very competitive Executive MBA ranked #12th Business school program in W. P. Carey School of Business at Arizona State University. The outcome variable is binary (0/1): admit or not admit. The predictor variables of interest include student gender and whether or not the student had an undergraduate degree in business. Because the response variable is binary, we need to use a model that handles 0/1 outcome variables correctly. Also, because the number of students involved is small, we will need a procedure that can perform the estimation with a small sample size.

8.7.1 Description of the Data

The data for this exact logistic data analysis include the number of students admitted, the total number of applicants broken down by gender (the variable **GENDER**), and whether or not they had an undergraduate business degree (the variable **DEGREE**).

Gender	Degree	admit	Frequency
0	0	0	5
0	0	1	2
0	1	0	4
0	1	1	6
1	0	0	6
1	0	1	0
1	1	0	1
1	1	1	6

8.7.2 Clustering

Later we learned that these 30 students came from 4 companies (A = 5; B = 6; C = 9; D = 10). These companies have a working relationship with the school and will provide financial support for the students who are admitted. These companies are seen as clusters.

References

Connolly, M. A., & Liang, K. (1988). Conditional logistic regression models for correlated binary 527 data. *Biometrika, 75*(3), 501–506.

Corcoran, C. L., Ryan, P. S., Mehta, C., Patel, N., & Monenbergs, G. (2001). An exact trend test for correlated binary data. *Biometrika, 57*, 941–948.

Cox, D. R. (1970). *Analysis of binary data*. Metheun.

Derr, R. E. (2000). Performing exact logistic regression with the SAS system. In *Proceedings of the twenty-fifth annual SAS users group international conference*.

Forster, J. J., McDonald, J. W., & Smith, P. W. F. (2003). Markov chain Monte Carlo exact inference for binomial and multinomial logistic regression models. *Statistics and Computing, 13*, 169–177.

Jones, A., & Huddleston, E. (2009). *SAS/STAT 9.2 user's guide*. SAS Institute.

Mehta, C. R., & Patel, N. R. (1995). Exact logistic regression: Theory and examples. *Statistics in Medicine, 14*, 2143–2160.

Siegel, S. (1957). Nonparametric statistics. *The American Statistician, 11*(3), 13–19. 3.

Troxler, S., Lalonde, T., & Wilson, J. R. (2011). Exact logistic models for nested binary data. *Statistics in Medicine, 30*(8), 866–876.

Part III
Analyzing Correlated Data Through Systematic Components

Chapter 9
Two-Level Nested Logistic Regression Model

9.1 Motivating Example

9.1.1 Description of the Case Study

The subset of the *Medicare* data analyzed in earlier chapters concentrated on the chance of rehospitalization of 1625 patients on three different but successive occasions during 2003–2005. We revisit these data in this chapter, but we concentrate on methods that contribute to prediction for an individual. Recall, the CFO of a hospital wanted to know whether the total number of diagnoses, total number of procedures performed, length of stay during the previous stay, and whether the patient has coronary atherosclerosis have any impact on rehospitalization within 30 days of discharge. In considering these data about the patients' histories and characteristics, we suspect that patient outcomes may be affected in some way by their different characteristics as well as the repeated measures on an individual must have impact on future outcomes. In addition, there may be effects that are attributable to the individual patient. In other words, we may have some unmeasurable effects. We wish to take all these potential factors into account as we analyze these data for the ultimate time. We want to use our findings to make predictions about the possibility of rehospitalization.

9.1.2 Study Hypotheses

Though we addressed these data earlier, we revisit these data in this chapter since we believe that there are unobservable and unmeasurable effects that exist among the patients that could be attributed to their outcomes. In particular, we want the probability of whether a patient with certain characteristics is rehospitalized in

J. R. Wilson et al., *Modeling Binary Correlated Responses*, ICSA Book Series in Statistics, https://doi.org/10.1007/978-3-031-62427-8_9

30 days. Using these measurements, we wish to identify the impact of the covariates on the rehospitalization. There are the individual's unobservable effects in this analysis of the data, as such one needs a subject-specific model as opposed to a marginal model as we did in Chap. 6 based on the GEE model. The GEE model looks at adjusting the variance in the random component to address the correlation, but in this chapter, we will introduce random effects into the systematic component to address the correlation. These two different approaches address, GEE and subject specifics, answer two different questions. One is the probability of the average outcome, while the other is the probability of an individual outcome. Based on our fitted models and analysis, if the unobservable effects among patients are not different, then the two models will give the same results.

9.2 Definition and Notation

A *generalized linear mixed model* is considered an extension of the generalized linear model (Chap. 3 with independent observations), in which the linear predictor contains random effects in addition to the fixed effects. It is called a "mixed" model because it addresses fixed and random effects at the same time.

Random effects are the unobservable differential effects among clusters. They are useful in avoiding erroneous conclusions (Hox & Maas, 2002). They are used to estimate population variance and include sampling variation (McCulloch, 2003). They consist of a sample of items from a large population that have varying effects on the response. They are therefore unobservable but believed to belong to a population with a certain mean and variance. They are used to address clustering, spatial correlation, and other forms of dependence among outcomes and are usually assumed to be normally distributed (Wolfinger, 1993). Our interest is in their variance. If the variance is estimated to be different from zero, we interpret this to mean that there are differential effects across individuals or clusters.

The *fixed effects* are those that assume no sampling error or random variance. They are the only factors of interest (Allison, 1999), and our interest is in their means.

A *random intercept model* is a model in which intercept (or constant term) is allowed to vary based on a certain distribution. Thus, the scores of the dependent variable for each individual observation differ based on an intercept with an assumed distribution. This distribution on the intercept is what distinguishes one from another. Our interest is in the means. Top-right image above showing the slope is consistent across individuals or clusters, but the starting point (intercept) changes.

A *random slope model* is a model in which the slopes are allowed to vary, and therefore, the slopes are different across groups. It implies that the slope, based on a certain variable, follows a certain distribution. Our interest is in the means. Bottom-left image above shows a common starting point (intercept), but the rate-of-change (slope) is different across individuals or clusters. Figure 9.1 gives a schematic diagram between fixed and random models.

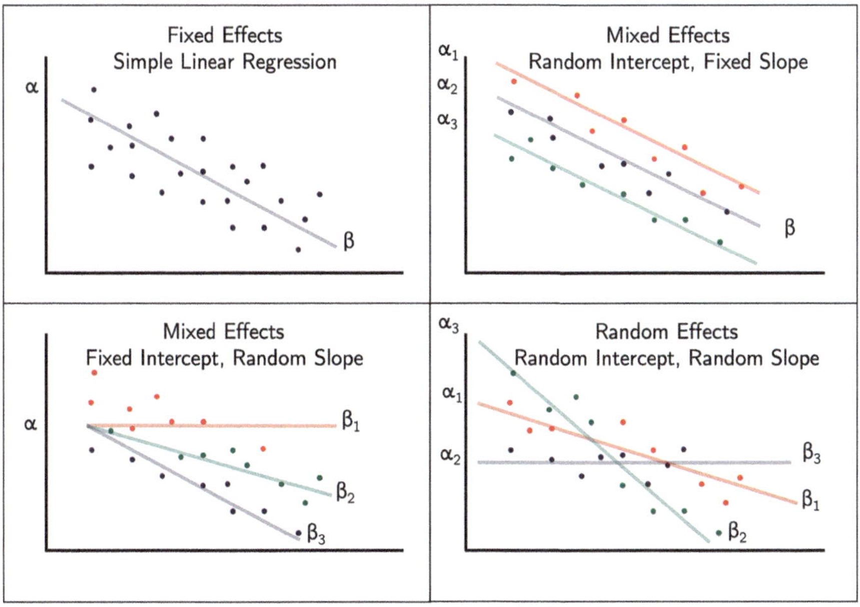

Fig. 9.1 Mixed models. (Image source: https://bookdown.org/steve_midway/DAR/random-effects.html)

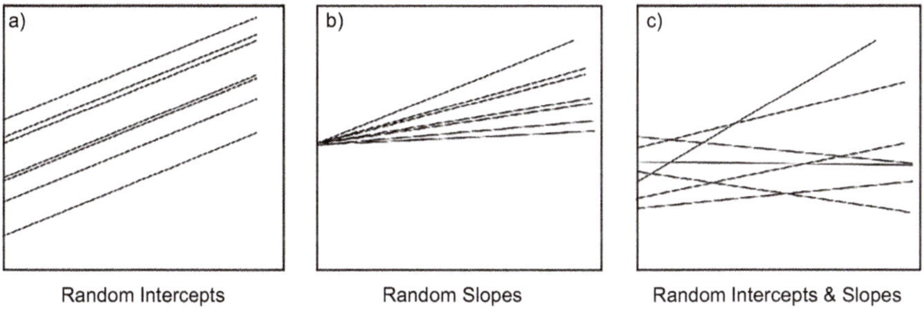

Fig. 9.2 Graphical insight into random slope models. (Image source: Fernée & Trimmis, 2021)

A *random intercept and slope model* is a model that includes both random intercepts and random slopes and is likely to be the most realistic type of models, although it is also the most complex. In this model, both intercepts and slopes are allowed to vary across groups. Thus, they are allowed to take certain shapes and values free of any common presumption. Bottom-right image above showing both the starting point and rate-of-change (intercept and slope) are different across individuals or clusters.

Figure 9.2 Image highlighting models producing plots with random intercepts but a common slope (a), random slopes but a common intercept (b), and random intercepts and slopes (c)

Quadrature is the process of dividing something into small squares. It is a technique for finding the area of a nonlinear surface. It involves the construction of a square with an area equal to that of a specified surface.

9.3 Exploratory Analyses

Let us consider a simple approach to these data based on intuition and an assumed knowledge of standard logistic regression. We fit a logistic regression model for each time period that the patient was in the hospital based on the length of stay (LOS) predictors. It results in three logistic regression models. We notice that these models are essentially different. This suggests that there are factors other than LOS working to influence rehospitalization within 30 days. We fit 1625 logistic regression models, one for each patient (cluster). It suggests that not all patients have the same factors contributing to hospitalization. Each patient provides certain effects, whether negative or positive relative to other patients, and as such must be accounted for. We propose that the repeatedness within each patient provides certain effects whether negative or positive relative to other patients and as such must be accounted for. These are the so-called random effects. In this chapter, we fit a two-way nested-level logistic regression model.

The generalized linear mixed model is an extension of the generalized linear model in that the linear predictor contains random effects in addition to the fixed effects. As such, the model gives rise to subject-specific or individual types of interpretations. The generalized linear mixed model presents the conditional probabilities rather than the marginal probabilities. While one chooses to use indicator variables to denote the categorical variable (patient), there are certain disadvantages with that indicator variable approach. In particular, in such a case, there are 1625–1 = 1624 indicator variables, thus resulting in a large number of parameters (indicator variables) in the model. In such a case, our results are applicable to the 1625 patients we sampled.

A generalized linear mixed model is depicted in Fig. 9.3, which shows a set of three types of X variables (X_A, X_B, X_C) as well as two Z variables (Z_A, Z_R). The X variables are continuous (X_A), categorical (X_B), and binary X_C but represent the fixed effects. Alternatively, the Z variables (Z_A, Z_R) denote the random effects, where both X and Z variables are impacting the variation in the response variable Y. The response variable is repeated measured on unit i (y_i: $y_{i1}, y_{i2}, \ldots\ldots, y_{iT}$). While generalized linear models (no Z variables) specify a distribution of the responses, generalized linear mixed models (X, Z) specify a distribution for the conditional response (Breslow & Clayton, 1993). When observations exhibit some form of dependency, such as with measurements taken from the same experimental unit or observations collected over time, hierarchical situations, clustered structures, or more commonly nested sources of variability, it is appropriate to fit a generalized linear mixed model.

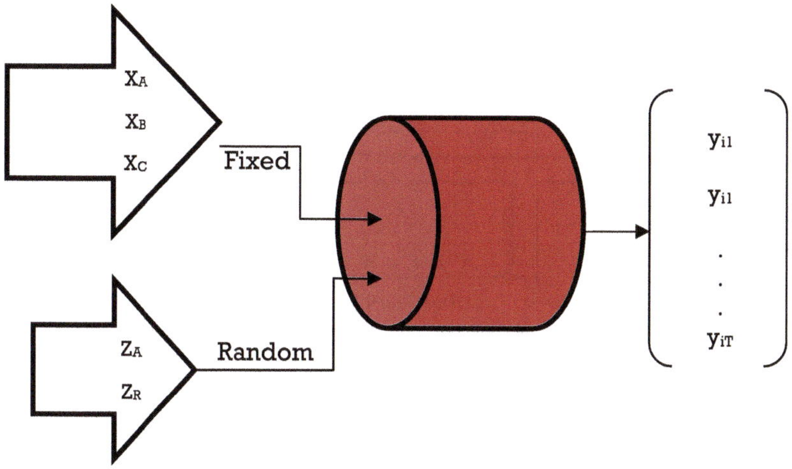

Fig. 9.3 Depicting a generalized linear mixed model

If we were to use the standard logistic regression model to analyze correlated data (where the repeated observations are affected by a common mechanism), it results in statistical inferences that are not accurate. In addition, we fit two correlated models. One is the conditional model and the other is a marginal model. In this chapter, we demonstrate the two models and show they are addressing different hypotheses.

9.3.1 Medicare

When the *Medicare* data were analyzed in Chap. 6 using GEE, the correlation among responses per patient was accounted for in the random component. However, in this chapter, we analyze the data accounting for the correlation through the systematic component. In Chaps. 6 and 7, we fitted marginal models to show the probability of rehospitalization, whereas in this chapter, we will fit subject-specific models and therefore model the probability of rehospitalization, given the random effect. The dataset used for this analysis has complete information for 1625 patients, and each patient has three outcomes (time from discharge to rehospitalized greater than 30 days), indicating four different times of rehospitalization. We can think of these as "times or occasions" nested within each patient (see Fig. 9.4).

These kinds of data lend themselves to a set of models that are sometimes referred to as mixed models, multilevel models, random coefficient models, or variance component models (Breslow & Clayton, 1993; Longford, 1993; Hox, 2002; Goldstein, 2003). We refer to them as generalized linear mixed models in this book.

Specifically, we present the nested logistic regression model as it pertains to allowing one random effect, which is equivalent to a two-level nested logistic

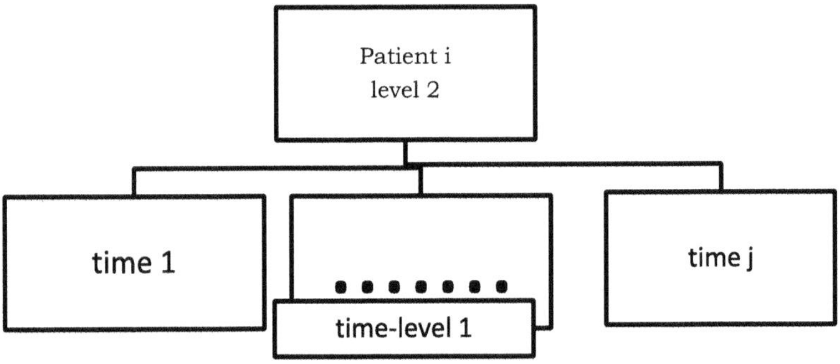

Fig. 9.4 Hierarchical structure for two levels

regression model. We fit the nested logistic regression model with both PROC NLMIXED and PROC GLIMMIX in SAS, as well as in SPSS, R, and STATA. We fit both the random intercept model and the random intercept and random slope model.

9.4 Statistical Model

Studies including repeated measures are expected to give rise to correlated data. Such types of data are common in many disciplines, including healthcare, banking, poll tracking, and education. Subjects, or units, are followed over time and are repeatedly observed under different experimental conditions or are observed in clusters. Oftentimes, such data are available in hierarchical structures consisting of a subset of a population of units at several levels. For our analysis of the Medicare data, we use a method that includes the clustering effect accounted for directly into the model, unlike in Chaps. 4 and 6, where the clustering effect was virtually ignored. We analyze these data and test hypotheses based on a method that belongs to the class of generalized linear mixed models. The basic idea behind generalized linear mixed models is conceptually straightforward (McCulloch, 2003). It incorporates random effects into the systematic component of a generalized linear model to account for the sampling. As such, it allows one to model correlation in the context of a broad class of models with non-normally distributed responses. These models are most useful when we account for both fixed and random effects in the model. This method of analyzing the data does not necessarily answer the same question as in Chap. 6.

The generalized linear mixed model is a specific type of statistical model. It belongs to a larger family of which generalized linear model is a special case. It is used to analyze correlated data and allows for non-normal data with random effects as well as correlation among responses. It is an extension of the class of generalized linear models. It allows normally distributed random effects and incorporates random effects into the linear predictor as part of the systematic component (McCulloch, 2003).

9.4.1 Marginal and Conditional Models

Whenever we talk about random effects, it is important to make clear the distinction between marginal and conditional models. It is not often that one speaks of the comparisons between marginal and random effects models. However, it is important to note that they do not measure the same thing. One measures or predicts the marginal probability and the other measures or predicts the conditional probability. To assist in clarifying this important distinction, consider the following situation with a sample of J hospitals each with n_{ij} patients: j = 1,…,J. We are interviewing these patients to measure whether or not their satisfaction with their hospital-stay differs based on whether or not the patient has signed up for a new healthcare plan. Consider fitting the *marginal* logistic model:

$$\log\left(\frac{P_{ij}}{1-P_{ij}}\right) = \beta_0 + \beta_1 H_{c=1}$$

where P_{ij} is the probability of $Y_{ij} = 1$ (the event, whether the patient is satisfied or not) and $H_{c=1}$ denotes whether or not they signed up. Then, $\mathrm{var}(y_{ij}) = P_{ij}(1 - P_{ij})$ and $\mathrm{cov}(y_{ij}, y_{ij}) = \alpha$. This is a marginal model that tells us about healthcare status and satisfaction, but it ignores the hospitals to which the patient belongs. If we want to talk about only the J hospitals in the sample, we add a series of J-1 binary variables to account for the specific hospital. This requires J-1 extra parameters, and one would not be able to say anything about the hospitals that are not represented in our sample. Because this sums over the hospitals, it is a marginal model.

Let us consider the *random effects* logistic model,

$$\log\left(\frac{p_s}{p_{ns}} | \gamma_j\right) = \beta_0 + \beta_1 H_{c=1} + \gamma_j$$

where γ_j denotes the differential effects among hospitals considered to be rescaled to a mean of zero, with $\gamma_j \sim N(0, \delta^2)$ as distributed as normal with mean zero and variance δ^2. The random intercept γ_j represents the combined effect of all omitted subject-specific covariates that cause some outcomes to be more prone to the event versus non-event. In this model, the correlation is due to the fact that patients in the same hospital share similar experiences. Once we have accounted for the hospital, in other words, given the hospital, we have eliminated the common difference, so we assume that the observations are independent. The marginal model assumes that the impact of a patient's healthcare status on satisfaction is the same across hospitals, whereas the random effects model tells us about what is expected in terms of patient satisfaction for each hospital. It is a conditional model, meaning the satisfaction of patients is conditional on which hospital in which they receive treatment. Because the patients do not answer the same question or model the same probability, we can refer to a marginal or population-averaged model and also to a subject-specific model. Using a set of binary variables to introduce the hospital factor leads to a number of additional parameters, leading one to use a fixed effects model since the results are restricted to the hospital observed. However, the use of the random intercept model measures the differences between hospitals and extends the conclusions made to hospitals that are not in the data.

The key distinction lies in the fact that the logistic regression models provide a nonlinear function on the probability scale, and the average of a nonlinear function is not the same as a linear function of the average. However, the relationship holds with linear functions where the regression coefficients in random effects models and marginal models are identical. Such is the case with regression models with identity link (meaning that the mean is related to the covariates with the identity function).

9.4.2 Two-Level Nested Logistic Regression with Random Intercept Model

The random intercept model is the simplest of the generalized linear mixed models. It augments the linear predictor with a single random effect for each unit:

$$\text{logit}\{\text{Prob of outcome}|\text{covariates}\} = \beta_0 + \beta_1 X_{ij1} + \ldots + \beta_P X_{ijP} + \gamma_i$$

where γ_i is the random effects associated with cluster *i*, which may represent a patient, for example, with repeated observations. So, differences among the patients are denoted by specific log odds ratio parameters.

In the Medicare data, the random effect pertains to the heterogeneity due to the patient *i*. So, instead of having a categorical variable representing the patients that only differentiate among patients in the data, we allow patients to be a subset of the population of patients and to have a different baseline but same rate of change over time. It allows each patient to have a different intercept but the same slope. These random effects represent the influence of the difference over time (units) on the outcomes that were not captured by the observed covariates. The random effect approach captures any unaccounted variation beyond the covariates in the data. Thus, the model is

$$\text{logit}\{\mu_{ij}|, X_{ij1} \ldots X_{ijP}|, \gamma_i\} = \beta_0 + \beta_1 X_{ij1} + \ldots + \beta_P X_{ijP} + \gamma_i$$

$$\gamma_i \sim \text{Normal}\left(0, \delta_\gamma^2\right)$$

where μ_{ij} is the mean of the distribution of the random component, β_i represents the regression coefficients, and the parameter δ_γ^2 indicates the variance in the population of random effect distribution and as such measures the degree of heterogeneity among patients (Blackwelder et al., 1998). We model the conditional distribution of the probability of outcome, given the random effects due to patients. Thus, we provide a conditional model in which we model the conditional mean of a binary response, given the random effects. We are modeling

$$g\left[E\left(y_{ij}|\gamma_i\right)\right]=g\left(\mu_{ij}\right)=\beta_0+\overbrace{\beta_1 X_{ij1}+\ldots+\beta_P X_{ijP}}+\overbrace{\gamma_i}.$$

We specify a distribution for the conditional response $y_{ij} \mid \gamma_i$ and a distribution for γ_i. As such, we present two parts, the random variation for the conditional part that we refer to as the R-side and the random variation for the distribution of the random effects that we refer to as the G-side. The R-side is due to the random component, while the G-side terms are in the systematic component. The G-side effects are inside the link function and are thus interpretable. In addition, we talk about the R-side random effect, which is what we retain when no random effects are in the model $\{+\beta_1 X_{ij1} + \ldots + \beta_P X_{ijP}\}$. R-side effects are outside the link function and, as such, are considered more difficult to interpret. When there is a G- and R-side, we refer to this as a generalized linear mixed model or as a subject-specific model. When there is no G-side, but only R-side, we refer to this as a marginal model that is a generalized linear model. In such a case, we are modeling the expected value of the outcome E(Y) (Dean & Nielsen, 2007; Have et al., 1999). The observations have the same correlation for given covariate values regardless of the cluster to which these observations belong.

9.4.3 *Interpretation of Parameter Estimates*

An important consideration for this type of model is how to interpret unobserved γ_i. When $\gamma_i = 0$, we consider all effects as zero. We can think of γ_i as unmeasured covariates or as a way to model heterogeneity in the correlated data. We can interpret β_0 as the log odds of $y_{ij} = 1$ when $X_{ij1} = 0$ and $\gamma_i = 0$; β_1 is the effect on the log odds for a unit increase in X_{ij1} for individuals in the same group, which will have the same value of γ_i. We can look at γ_i as the effect of being in group *i* or the residual at level *i*. The $[\beta_1 \ldots ., \beta_P]$ parameters are referred to as cluster specific or patient-specific of X_{ij1}.

To interpret the coefficient β_1, we can keep the subject-specific latent effect γ_{0i} the same and let the covariate change from X_1 to $X_1 + 1$.

$$\text{logit}\left(\text{Prob of rehospitalization}|\text{patient}\right)=\beta_0+\beta_1\left(X_1+1\right)+\beta_2 X_2+\gamma_{0i} \quad \text{minus}$$

$$\text{logit}\left(\text{Prob of rehospitalization}|\text{patient}\right)=\beta_0+\beta_1 X_1+\beta_2 X_2+\gamma_{0i}=\beta_1.$$

Then, the difference in logit is β_1. So, in order to make comparisons, as we did with the standard logistic regression, we must keep the random effects the same.

Therefore, patients with the same random effects and same X_2 are exp. (β_1) times more likely to be rehospitalized if they are $(X_1 + 1)$ as opposed to X_1.

The exponent β_i $(e^{\beta i})$ is an odds ratio, comparing odds for patients one unit different on X_{ij1}, but in the same group. The response probability for individual i in group j calls for some values for γ_i. Larsen et al. (2000) discussed that conditioning on the random effects yields the same nice interpretation in terms of odds ratios as in the case of ordinary logistic regression models. However, it is not necessarily possible to condition on unobservable random effects. The odds ratio is a random variable rather than a fixed parameter and as such should be kept in mind when interpreting the model.

Observations within a cluster are assumed to be independent given the random cluster effect (conditional independence). Thus, we get the product of the conditional probabilities across the time points within a cluster to yield the conditional probability. These models are fit by maximizing the product of conditional probabilities over cluster i and the marginal likelihood for cluster i. We rely on numerical integration achieved by working with approximations for the product of integrals. In particular, we have a combination of a binomial distribution as the conditional distribution and a normal distribution for the random effects. The joint distribution involves a procedure that allows integrating out the random effects but that is very tedious so instead we rely on the conditional distribution.

9.4.4 *Two-Level Nested Logistic Regression Model with Random Intercept and Slope*

In the two-level nested logistic regression model with random intercepts, we are assuming that the rate of change remains the same for each patient (cluster). Now, consider the following model:

$$\text{logit}\left(P_1|,\gamma_0|,\gamma_1\right) = \beta_0 + \beta_1 X_1 + \beta_2 X_2 + \gamma_{0i} + \gamma_{1i} Z_1$$

where γ_{0i} is distributed as normal with a mean of zero and the variance $\delta^2_{\gamma 0}$ and γ_{1i} is distributed as normal with a mean of zero and variance $\delta^2_{\gamma 1}$ (Schabenberger, 2005). This model assumes that, given γ_{0i} and γ_{1i}, the responses from the same cluster are mutually independent or, rather, that the correlation between units from the same cluster is completely explained by them having been in the same cluster. As such, these are called subject-specific parameter models (Hu et al., 1998). Each cluster has its own intercept and slope. In the random intercept model, we assumed that these intercepts have a normal distribution with mean zero and variance $\delta^2_{\gamma 0}$. The model assumes that each cluster starts at a different point and changes at different rates. However, if that variance is found to be different from zero, then we conclude that there is a need for assuming different intercepts. Similarly, we assume that the rate of change over a particular random effect has a normal distribution with mean zero and variance $\delta_{\gamma 1}^2$.

9.5 Analysis of Data

We used the two-level nested logistic regression model with random intercepts (*Model 1*) and the two-level nested logistic regression model with both random intercepts and random slopes (*Model 2*) to analyze the Medicare data. We used PROC NLMIXED and PROC GLIMMIX in SAS and also used SPSS R and STATA. We used the three periods of complete data and treated the patients as clusters with random effects. Thus, time is nested within each patient.

9.5.1 Two-Level Nested Logistic Regression Model with Random Intercepts Using SAS (PROC NLMIXED Versus PROC GLIMMIX)

We can fit generalized linear mixed models with PROC NLMIXED and PROC GLIMMIX. There are several important differences between PROC NLMIXED and PROC GLIMMIX worth stating based on our experience, as shown in examples in this chapter and the next.

1. Both SAS procedures approach parameter estimation as an optimization problem.
2. Both SAS procedures are appropriate when the models are simple and limited to two levels, the number of random effects is small, and the number of level 2 groups is relatively large.
3. The PROC NLMIXED procedure is recommended for analysis of binary data that require accurate covariance parameter estimates, or for cases where nested models need to be compared.
4. PROC NLMIXED is superior for multilevel analysis involving small groups, such as family studies (Murray et al., 2004).
5. PROC NLMIXED delivers exact maximum likelihood estimates of the parameters if the number of quadrature points is large enough. We use this in Chap. 10.
6. The PROC NLMIXED procedure does not have a class statement, so the user must use indicator variables when faced with categorical variables.
7. For repeated binary responses with few repeated measures on each subject, PROC GLIMMIX can produce biased results (Breslow & Clayton, 1993).
8. PROC GLIMMMIX provides less accurate estimates and produces potentially biased estimates for both fixed effects and covariance parameters (Schabenberger, 2005).

Two-Level Nested Logistic Regression Model with Random Intercepts Using SAS (PROC GLIMMIX)

SAS Program Code

THE GLIMMIX PROCEDURE

We first present the use of PROC GLIMMIX to analyze these data. We present NDX, NPR, LOS, DX101, and the categorical variable time represented by T_2 and T_3. A partial presentation of the data is given in Table 9.1.

```
data mydata; set chapter9; run;
T2=(time=2); T3=(time=3);
title 'GLIMMIX with random intercept';
PROC GLIMMIX data=mydata method=quad;
CLASS PNUM_R;
model biRadmit(event = '1')=NDX NPR LOS DX101 T2 T3/DIST=BINARY
LINK=LOGIT DDFM=BW SOLUTION OR;
RANDOM INTERCEPT/ subject =PNUM_R;
run;
```

Comment The model statement provides results for the R-side with fixed effects. This takes care of the R-side with fixed effects. RANDOM statement denotes the parameter on which the random effects are associated. This takes care of the distribution of the random effects. This program code yields the following SAS output:

Table 9.1 Partial look of the medicare data

PNUM_R	biRadmit	NDX	NPR	LOS	DX101	time	T_2	T_3
127	0	9	6	6	1	1	0	0
127	0	6	4	1	1	2	1	0
127	0	9	5	3	1	3	0	1
560	1	9	3	8	0	1	0	0
560	0	9	1	17	0	2	1	0
560	0	7	1	6	0	3	0	1
746	1	6	4	12	0	1	0	0
746	0	6	1	1	0	2	1	0
746	0	9	1	2	0	3	0	1
750	0	9	3	6	0	1	0	0
750	1	7	3	4	0	2	1	0
750	1	9	2	4	0	3	0	1

SAS Output

```
                        THE GLIMMIX PROCEDURE
                         Model Information
Dataset                                  WORK.MYDATA
Response Variable                        biRadmit
Response Distribution                    Binary
Link Function                            Logit
Variance Function                        Default
Variance Matrix Blocked By               PNUM_R
Estimation Technique                     Maximum Likelihood
Likelihood Approximation                 Gauss-Hermite Quadrature
Degrees of Freedom Method                Between-Within
                        THE GLIMMIX PROCEDURE
Class Level Information
Class      Levels    Values
PNUM_R      1625     127 560 746 750 1117 1395 1568 2076 2390 2413
............ 1371713
```

Comment These are the cluster ID numbers. There are ID numbers through "PNUM_R." All 1625 were listed but were truncated for space issues.

```
Number of Observations Read         4875
Number of Observations Used         4875
```

Comment There are 4875 observations read as 1625 × 3 = 4875. Read and used are equal since the data are complete.

Response Profile

```
Ordered                      Total
Value     biRadmit           Frequency
1             0                 2433
2             1                 2442
The GLIMMIX procedure is modeling the probability that
biRadmit='1'.
```

Comment Each patient had 3 visits which is 1625*3 = 4875 observations. Of the 4875 observations, 2442 were rehospitalized within 30 days, given by biRadmit = '1'.

Dimensions

G-side Cov. Parameters	1
Columns in X	7
Columns in Z per Subject	1
Subjects (Blocks in V)	1625
Max Obs per Subject	3

Comment This (G-side cov.) is the variance of random effects. There are 7 fixed effects covariates (intercept, NDX, NPR, LOS, DX101, T_2, T_3). There was one random effect covariate in the G-side (columns in Z), as represented by random intercept. This (1625) represents the number of clusters. The maximum size of the clusters is three.

Optimization Information

Optimization Technique	Dual Quasi-Newton
Parameters in Optimization	8
Lower Boundaries	1
Upper Boundaries	0
Fixed Effects	Not Profiled
Starting From	GLM estimates
Quadrature Points	5

Comment Sometimes the model may not converge, and you will need to increase the quadrature points to get convergence as well as to get an estimate for the random effects variance and standard error.

THE GLIMMIX PROCEDURE

Iteration History

Objective Max

Iteration	Restarts	Evaluations	Function	Change	Gradient
0	0	4	6735.2172141	.	153.4744
1	0	4	6733.7716779	1.44553618	143.9054
2	0	5	6733.349135	0.42254286	141.7167
3	0	2	6667.5705532	65.77858185	507.3751
4	0	5	6652.2001902	15.37036297	206.4346
5	0	3	6644.4503699	7.74982030	264.8008
6	0	4	6621.9315943	22.51877565	117.7424
7	0	3	6618.9815278	2.95006646	35.97061
8	0	4	6618.81057	0.17095779	18.10109
9	0	2	6618.6997135	0.11085648	45.43903
10	0	3	6618.6591506	0.04056298	15.15351
11	0	4	6618.657243	0.00190758	2.848396
12	0	3	6618.6570395	0.00020348	1.052471
13	0	3	6618.6570292	0.00001034	0.1689

Convergence criterion (GCONV=1E-8) satisfied.

Comment The model converges and the coefficients are acceptable.

FIT STATISTICS

-2 Log Likelihood	6618.66
AIC (smaller is better)	6634.66
AICC (smaller is better)	6634.69
BIC (smaller is better)	6677.80
CAIC (smaller is better)	6685.80
HQIC (smaller is better)	6650.67

Comment These fit statistics are about the fit of the model. However, without a p-value, it is difficult to make a conclusion with these statistics. They are best suited if you are comparing nested models.

Fit Statistics for Conditional Distribution

-2 log L(biRadmit | r. effects)	6114.57
Pearson Chi-square	4479.14
Pearson Chi-square / DF	0.92

Comment The fit of the model is measured by generalized: Chi-square / DF = 0.92. This is usually compared to the value 1.0. The other two statistics, −2 log L(biRadmit | r. effects) and Pearson Chi-square, are also fit statistics for the conditional distribution. They tell about the conditional part of the model where the random effects are given.

Covariance Parameter Estimates

Cov Parm	Subject	Estimate	Standard Error
Intercept	PNUM_R	0.2525	0.07773

Comment The variance of the random effects is $(0.07773)^2$ and the estimate is 0.2525. Thus, the standardized value is 0.2525/0.07773 = 3.248, which suggests that there is heterogeneity among the patients (clusters). The random effects are significant. It was prudent to have differential effects among the patients.

Solutions For Fixed Effects

Effect	Estimate	Standard Error	DF	t Value	Pr > |t|
Intercept	-0.3933	0.1351	1624	-2.91	0.0037
NDX	0.07056	0.01655	3244	4.26	<.0001
NPR	-0.02789	0.01979	3244	-1.41	0.1587
LOS	0.03267	0.005827	3244	5.61	<.0001
DX101	-0.1413	0.09749	3244	-1.45	0.1474
T_2	-0.4086	0.07401	3244	-5.52	<.0001
T_3	-0.2528	0.07433	3244	-3.40	0.0007

Comment The conditional model is

$$\log\left(\hat{P}_{y=1} \,|\, \hat{P}_{y=0}\right) = -0.393 + 0.071\text{NDX} - 0.028\text{NPR} + 0.033\text{LOS}$$
$$-0.141\text{DX101} - 0.409\text{T}_2 - 0.253\text{T}_3$$

$$\frac{Odds\left(\text{y} = 1|\text{NDX} = \text{n}+1, \text{NPR} = 0, \text{LOS} = \text{p}, \text{DX101} = 0, T_2 = 0, T_3 = 0, \text{for patient j}\right)}{Odds\left(\text{y} = 1|\text{NDX} = \text{n}, \text{NPR} = 0, \text{LOS} = \text{p}, \text{DX101} = 0, T_2 = 0, T_3 = 0, \text{for patient j}\right)}$$
$$= \exp\left(\beta_{NDX}\right) = \exp\left(0.0706\right)$$

The odds of rehospitalization per NDX for each patient with no coronary atherosclerosis is exp (0.0706)=1.073. The odds of rehospitalization per NDX for each patient with coronary atherosclerosis and all other things equal are exp. (0.0706–0.1413)=0.932. The odds decrease by 7% for patients with coronary atherosclerosis. The fixed effects, based on the added effects given other covariates, show that NDX ($p < 0.0001$) and LOS ($p < 0.0001$) were significant.

Odds Ratio Estimates

NDX	NPR	LOS	DX101	T2	T3	_NDX	_NPR	_LOS	_DX101	_T_2	_T_3
8.466	2.827	5.913	0.1485	0.333	0.333	**7.467**	2.827	5.913	0.1485	0.333	0.333
7.466	**3.827**	5.913	0.1485	0.333	0.333	7.467	**2.828**	5.913	0.1485	0.333	0.333
7.466	2.827	**6.913**	0.1485	0.333	0.333	7.467	2.828	**5.913**	0.1485	0.333	0.333
7.466	2.827	5.913	**1.1485**	0.333	0.333	7.467	2.828	5.913	**0.1485**	0.333	0.333
7.466	2.827	5.913	0.1485	**1.333**	0.333	7.467	2.828	5.913	0.1485	**0.333**	0.333
7.466	2.827	5.913	0.1485	0.333	**1.333**	7.467	2.828	5.913	0.1485	0.333	**0.333**

The effects of continuous variables are assessed as one unit offset from the mean. The AT suboption modifies the reference value and the UNIT suboption modifies the offsets.

Odds Ratio Estimates

NDX	NPR	LOS	DX101	T2	T3	_NDX	_NPR	_LOS	_DX101	_T2	Estimate
8.466	2.827	5.913	0.1485	0.333	0.333	7.467	2.828	5.913	0.149	0.333	**1.073**
7.466	3.827	5.913	0.1485	0.333	0.333	7.467	2.828	5.913	0.149	0.333	**0.972**
7.466	2.827	6.913	0.1485	0.333	0.333	7.467	2.828	5.913	0.149	0.333	**1.033**
7.466	2.827	5.913	1.1485	0.333	0.333	7.467	2.828	5.913	0.149	0.333	**0.868**
7.466	2.827	5.913	0.1485	1.333	0.333	7.467	2.828	5.913	0.149	0.333	**0.665**
7.466	2.827	5.913	0.1485	0.333	1.333	7.467	2.828	5.913	0.149	0.333	**0.777**

The effects of continuous variables are assessed as one-unit offsets from the mean. The AT suboption modifies the reference value and the UNIT suboption modifies the offsets.

Comment The estimate of the odds ratio are 1.073, 0.972, 1.033, 0.868, 0.665, and 0.777 for exp. (0.07056); exp. (−0.02789); exp. (0.03267); exp.(−0.1413); exp. (−0.4086); and exp.(−0.2528) for NDX, NPR, LOS, DX101, T_2, and T_3, respectively.

Odds Ratio Estimates

NDX	NPR	LOS	DX101	T_2	T_3	_NDX	_NPR	_LOS	_DX101	_T2	DF
8.466	2.827	5.913	0.1485	0.333	0.3333	7.467	2.828	5.913	0.1485	0.333	3244
7.466	3.827	5.913	0.1485	0.333	0.333	7.467	2.828	5.913	0.1485	0.333	3244
7.466	2.827	6.913	0.1485	0.333	0.333	7.467	2.828	5.913	0.1485	0.333	3244

The effects of continuous variables are assessed as one-unit offsets from the mean. The AT suboption modifies the reference value and the UNIT suboption modifies the offsets.

Odds Ratio Estimates

NDX	NPR	LOS	DX101	T2	T3	_NDX	_NPR	_LOS	_DX101	_T2	DF
7.466	2.827	5.913	1.1485	0.333	0.333	7.467	2.828	5.913	0.1485	0.333	3244
7.466	2.827	5.913	0.1485	1.333	0.333	7.467	2.828	5.913	0.1485	0.333	3244
7.466	2.827	5.913	0.1485	0.333	1.333	7.467	2.828	5.913	0.1485	0.333	3244

The effects of continuous variables are assessed as one-unit offsets from the mean. The AT suboption modifies the reference value and the UNIT suboption modifies the offsets.

Odds Ratio Estimates 95% Confidence

NDX	NPR	LOS	DX101	T2	T3	_NDX	_NPR	_LOS	_DX101	_T2	Limits
8.466	2.827	5.913	0.1485	0.333	0.333	7.467	2.828	5.913	0.1485	0.333	1.039
7.466	3.827	5.913	0.1485	0.333	0.333	7.467	2.828	5.913	0.1485	0.333	0.935
7.466	2.827	6.913	0.1485	0.333	0.333	7.467	2.828	5.913	0.1485	0.333	1.021
7.466	2.827	5.913	1.1485	0.333	0.333	7.467	2.828	5.913	0.1485	0.333	0.717
7.466	2.827	5.913	0.1485	1.333	0.333	7.4667	2.828	5.913	0.1485	0.333	0.575
7.466	2.827	5.913	0.1485	0.3333	1.333	7.467	2.828	5.913	0.1485	0.333	0.671

The effects of continuous variables are assessed as one-unit offsets from the mean. The AT suboption modifies the reference value and the UNIT suboption modifies the offsets.

Comment The lower limit of the odds ratio is given here.

Odds Ratio Estimates 95% Confidence

NDX	NPR	LOS	DX101	T2	T3	_NDX	_NPR	_LOS	_DX101	_T2	Limits
8.466	2.827	5.913	0.1485	0.333	0.333	7.467	2.828	5.913	0.1485	0.333	1.109
7.466	3.827	5.913	0.1485	0.333	0.333	7.467	2.828	5.913	0.1485	0.333	1.011
7.466	2.827	6.913	0.1485	0.333	0.333	7.467	2.828	5.913	0.1485	0.333	1.045
7.466	2.827	5.913	1.1485	0.333	0.333	7.467	2.828	5.913	0.1485	0.333	1.051
7.466	2.827	5.913	0.1485	1.333	0.333	7.467	2.828	5.913	0.1485	0.333	0.768
7.466	2.827	5.913	0.1485	0.333	1.333	7.467	2.828	5.913	0.1485	0.333	0.898

The effects of continuous variables are assessed as one-unit offsets from the mean. The AT suboption modifies the reference value and the UNIT suboption modifies the offsets.

Comment The upper limit of the odds ratio is given here.

TYPE III TESTS OF FIXED EFFECTS

Effect	Num DF	Den DF	F Value	Pr > F
NDX	1	3244	18.17	<.0001
NPR	1	3244	1.99	0.1587
LOS	1	3244	31.44	<.0001
DX101	1	3244	2.10	0.1474
T_2	1	3244	30.49	<.0001
T_3	1	3244	11.57	0.0007

Comment NDX and LOS show a significant impact on rehospitalization. The periods 2 and 3 are significantly different from period 1. The probability of being rehospitalized within 30 days the second or third time seems to be lower with each subsequent return.

Two-Level Nested Logistic Regression Model with Random Intercepts Using SAS (PROC NLMIXED)

Proc Nlmixed

The use of PROC NLMIXED for higher levels is important to later chapters. We present PROC NLMIXED here for comparison with PROC GLIMMIX and as a stepping stone to Chap. 10 when we analyze multi-levels.

```
TITLE 'NLMIXED WITH RANDOM INTERCEPT';
PROC NLMIXED DATA=MYDATA;
PARMS b0=-0.3675 b1=0.0648 b2=-0.0306 b3=0.0344 b4=-0.1143
b5=-0.3876 b6=-0.2412;
```

Comment To run NLMIXED, values for the coefficients must first be selected carefully in order to ensure convergence. We usually start with the estimates from GEE.

```
ETA=U+b0+b1*NDX+b2*NPR+b3*LOS+b4*DX101+b5*T2+b6*T3;
```

Comment This is the right-hand side of the systematic function.

```
EXPETA=EXP(ETA);
Comment: This is the link function.
P=(EXPETA/(1+EXPETA));
Comment: This is the probability on the probability scale.
MODEL BIRADMIT ~ BINARY (P);
RANDOM M ~ NORMAL (0, SIGMAU*SIGMAU) SUBJECT=PNUM_R;
```

Comment The random effects and their distribution are now incorporated. PARMS lists names of parameters and specifies initial values. Choosing adequate and precise initial parameter estimates promotes convergence. Parameters not listed in PARMS statement are assigned an initial value of 1. *Random* defines the random effects and their distribution. The only distribution currently available for the random effects is normal$(0, \delta^2)$. The *subject* = PNUM_R determines when new realizations of the random effects are assumed to occur. The input dataset should be clustered according to this variable.

```
RUN;
```

SAS Output

```
                         THE NLMIXED PROCEDURE
Specifications
Dataset                                        WORK.MYDATA
Dependent Variable                              biRadmit
Distribution for Dependent Variable             Binary
Random Effects                                  U
Distribution for Random Effects                 Normal
Subject Variable                                PNUM_R
Optimization Technique                          Dual Quasi-Newton
Integration Method                              Adaptive Gaussian
Quadrature
Dimensions
Observations Used                               4875
Observations Not Used                           0
Total Observations                              4875
Subjects                                        1625
Max Obs Per Subject                             3
Parameters                                      8
Quadrature Points                               5
Parameters
b0      b1      b2      b3      b4 b5     b6      SIGMAU  NegLogLike
-0.368 0.065  -0.031  0.034  -0.114   -0.388  -0.241  1  3336.808
```

Comment It provides the starting values for the beta coefficients and the variance of the random effects. Quadratures can be adjusted to help with convergence.

Iteration History

Iter	Calls	NegLogLike	Diff	MaxGrad	Slope
1	4	3335.05945	1.748835	172.6995	-867.441
2	7	3334.01585	1.0436	277.225	-2032.36
.					
11	25	3309.32852	0.000179	0.344287	-0.00041
12	27	3309.32851	7.854E-6	0.118542	-0.00002

GCONV convergence criterion satisfied.

Comment To know that you have convergence is important but not always possible. At times, you may need to adjust the number of quadrature points to facilitate convergence.

FIT STATISTICS

-2-Log-Likelihood	6618.7
AIC (smaller is better)	6634.7
AICC (smaller is better)	6634.7
BIC (smaller is better)	6677.8

Comment These are fit statistics that really cannot tell us if the model is a good fit.

PARAMETER ESTIMATES

Parameter	Estimate	Standard Error	DF	t Value	Pr > |t|	Alpha	Lower	Upper	Gradient
b0	-0.393	0.135	1624	-2.91	0.0037	0.05	-0.658	-0.1282	0.0035
b1	0.071	0.017	1624	4.26	<.0001	0.05	0.0381	0.103	0.0339
b2	-0.028	0.020	1624	-1.41	0.159	0.05	-0.067	0.011	-0.0116
b3	0.033	0.006	1624	5.61	<.0001	0.05	0.021	0.044	-0.1185
b4	-0.141	0.097	1624	-1.45	0.148	0.05	-0.333	0.050	0.001
b5	-0.410	0.074	1624	-5.52	<.0001	0.05	-0.554	-0.264	-0.001
b6	-0.253	0.074	1624	-3.40	0.0007	0.05	-0.399	-0.107	0.003
SIGMAU	0.502	0.077	1624	6.50	<.0001	0.05	0.351	0.654	0.0008

Comment The parameters take on the names b0, b1, b2, b3, b4, b5, and b6. The order follows the way they were presented in the systematic component. NDX (b1) and LOS (b3) are significant. The results are similar to those obtained with PROC GLIMMIX.

$$\log\left(\hat{P}_{y=1} \mid \hat{P}_{y=0}\right) = -0.393 + 0.071\text{NDX} - 0.028\text{NPR} + 0.033\text{LOS}$$
$$-0.141\text{DX101} - 0.410\text{T}_2 - 0.253\text{T}_3$$

$$\frac{Odds\left(\text{y} = 1 \mid \text{NDX} = \text{n}+1, \text{NPR} = 0, \text{LOS} = \text{p}, \text{DX101} = 0, T_2 = 0, T_3 = 0, \text{for patient j}\right)}{Odds\left(\text{y} = 1 \mid \text{NDX} = \text{n}, \text{NPR} = 0, \text{LOS} = \text{p}, \text{DX101} = 0, T_2 = 0, T_3 = 0, \text{for patient j}\right)}$$
$$= \exp\left(\beta_{NDX}\right) = \exp(0.071)$$

9.5.2 Two-Level Nested Logistic Regression Model with Random Intercepts Using SPSS

SPSS Model 1: Logistic Regression Model with random Intercepts

SPSS program

We fit the two-level logistic regression model with random intercepts using SPSS.

SPSS Pull Down Menu

Step 1:
In the data editor window select "Variable View" in the bottom left corner.
Make sure the following variables are set to the following "Measure":

1. PNUM_R ➔ Nominal (NOTE this is different than Chap. 6)
2. biRadmit ➔ Nominal
3. NDX ➔ Scale
4. NPR ➔ Scale
5. LOS ➔ Scale
6. DX101 ➔ Scale
7. T2 ➔ Nominal
8. T3 ➔ Nominal

Step 2:

Click "Analyze" on the toolbar
Select "Mixed Models"
Click "Generalized Linear"

Step 3:

Click the first tab labeled "Data Structure"
Select the subject variable in the left column
Drag the subject variable to the area under "Subjects" in the "Canvas:" area

Step 4:

Click the second tab labeled "Fields & Effects"
Select "Target" in the left column
Under "Target" in the right column, select "Use custom target"
Select the dependent variable from the pull down menu under "Target:"
Select "Binary logistic regression" under "Target Distribution…".

Step 5:

Select "Fixed Effects" in the left column
Select the independent variable and drag them under "Main" in the "Effect builder:" area

Step 6:

Select "Random Effects" in the left column
Click "Add Block" near the bottom

Step 6–1:

In the Add Block window click the check box next to "Include intercept"
Under "Subject combination" select PNUM_R
If performing the random intercept analysis only then click "OK"
If performing the random intercept and random slope for LOS analysis drag LOS from the left column to the area under "Main" and then click "OK"

Step 7:

Click the third tab labeled "Build Options"
Under "Sorting Order" select "Descending" for both options
Click "Run" near the bottom of the window

The SPSS procedure presents the following output.

SPSS output
Fixed Coefficients
Target: biRadmit
Reference category: 0

Model term	Coefficient	Std. error	t	Sig.	Lower	Upper
Intercept	−0.372	0.130	−2.861	0.004	−0.626	−0.117
NDX	0.066	0.016	4.181	0.000	0.035	0.097
NPR	−0.028	0.019	−1.462	0.144	−0.065	0.009
LOS	0.032	0.006	5.709	0.000	0.021	0.043
DX101	−0.128	0.094	−1.365	0.172	−0.311	0.056
T2 = 1	−0.388	0.072	−5.403	0.000	−0.529	−0.247
T3 = 1	−0.240	0.072	−3.327	0.001	−0.382	−0.099

Probability distribution: binomial
Link function: logit
This coefficient is set to zero because it is redundant

Comment The fitted logistic regression model is.

$$\log\left(\hat{P}_{y=1} \mid \hat{P}_{y=0}\right) = -0.372 + 0.066\text{NDX} - 0.028\text{NPR} + 0.032\text{LOS} - 0.128\text{DX101} - 0.388\text{T}_2 - 0.240\text{T}_3$$

. The covariates, NDX, LOS, T_2 and T_3 are significant. The link is logit= $\log\left(\hat{P}_{y=1} \mid \hat{P}_{y=0}\right)$.

Covariance Parameters
Target: biRadmit

Covariance parameters	Residual effect	0
	Random effects	1
Design matrix columns	Fixed effects	9
	Random effects	1[a]
Common subjects		1625

Common subjects are based on the subject specifications for the residual and random effects and are used to chunk the data for better performance
[a]This is the number of columns per common subject

Random effect	Estimate	Std. error	Z	Sig.	95% confidence interval Lower upper	
Var(intercept)	0.158	0.054	2.906	0.004	0.080	0.310

Covariance structure: variance components
Subject Specification: PNUM_R

Comment The variance of the random effects lies between [0.080, 0.310] based on a 95% confidence level. There is variation among the patients in regard to rehospitalization. The significance difference is also shown through the p-value = 0.004.

9.5.3 Two-Level Nested Logistic Regression Model with Random Intercepts Using R

R Program

We fit the two-level logistic regression model with random intercepts using R.

```
Random intercept
> glmer.out=glmer(biRadmit ~ NDX + NPR + LOS + DX101 + T2 + T3 +
(1|PNUM_R), data=data1, family=binomial)
> summary(glmer.out)
```

Generalized linear mixed model fit by the Laplace approximation.

```
Formula: biRadmit ~ NDX + NPR + LOS + DX101 + T2 + T3 + (1
| PNUM_R)
Data: data1
 AIC          BIC          logLik          deviance
 6639         6691         -3311           6623
```

Random effects:

```
Groups Name                Variance          Std.Dev.
PNUM_R (Intercept)         0.17115           0.4137
```

Comment The standard deviation of the variance of the random effects is 0.4137.

Number of obs: 4875, groups: PNUM_R, 1625.

Fixed effects:

	Estimate	Std. error	z value	Pr(>|z|)	
(Intercept)	−0.386178	0.130272	−2.964	0.003033	**
NDX	0.068966	0.015915	4.333	1.47E-05	***
NPR	−0.028793	0.019114	−1.506	0.131971	
LOS	0.033239	0.005681	5.851	4.87E-09	***
DX101	−0.133469	0.093952	−1.421	0.155432	
T2	−0.4031	0.07192	−5.605	2.08E-08	***
T3	−0.249785	0.072377	−3.451	0.000558	***

Signif. codes: 0 '***' 0.001 '**' 0.01 '*' 0.05 '.' 0.1 '' 1

Comment The fitted logistic regression model is $\log\left(\hat{P}_{y=1} | \hat{P}_{y=0}\right) = -0.386 + 0.069\text{NDX} - 0.029\text{NPR} + 0.033\text{LOS} - 0.133\text{DX101} - 0.388T_2 - 0.240T_3$. The covariates, NDX, LOS, T_2 and T_3 are significant. The link is logit.

Correlation Of Fixed Effects

	(Intr)	NDX	NPR	LOS	DX101	T2
NDX	-0.812					
NPR	-0.285	-0.061				
LOS	0.114	-0.286	-0.262			
DX101	-0.156	0.145	-0.368	0.202		
T2	-0.272	-0.038	0.080	-0.036	0.039	
T3	-0.248	-0.073	0.094	-0.041	0.067	0.510

Number of Observations: 4875

Number of Groups: 1625

9.5.4 *Two-Level Nested Logistic Regression Model with Random Intercepts Using STATA*

STATA Program

```
. MELOGIT BIRADMIT NDX NPR LOS DX101 T2 T3, PNUM_R:,
COVARIANCE(UNSTRUCTURED)
FITTING FIXED EFFECTS MODEL:
MIXED-EFFECTS LOGISTIC REGRESSION   NUMBER OF OBS
=      4,875
GROUP VARIABLE: PNUM_R              NUMBER OF GROUPS  =     1,625
OBS PER GROUP:
MIN =         3
AVG =       3.0
MAX =         3
INTEGRATION METHOD: MVAGHERMITE     INTEGRATION PTS.  =         7
WALD CHI2(6)    =     108.10
LOG LIKELIHOOD = -3309.3931            PROB > CHI2    =    0.0000
BIRADMIT   COEFFICIENT  STD. ERR.  Z    P>Z    [95% CONF.
INTERVAL]
NDX       .0706733   .0165516  4.27  0.000   .0382328      .1031137
NPR      -.028227    .0197812 -1.43  0.154  -.0669974      .0105434
LOS        .0327217  .005827   5.62  0.000   .021301       .0441424
DX101    -.1367701   .0973854 -1.40  0.160  -.3276419      .0541018
T2       -.4085625   .0740032 -5.52  0.000  -.5536062     -.2635188
T3       -.2526163   .074327  -3.40  0.001  -.398296      -.1069365
_CONS     -.3941909   .1351169  -2.92 0.004  -.6590151    -.1293668
PNUM_R
VAR(_CONS) .252085  .0776874    .1377921     .4611793
LR TEST VS.LOGISTIC MODEL:CHIBAR2(01)=13.87 PROB >= CHIBAR2 = 0.0001
```

Comment The above correlation estimates and standard errors of the fixed effects match those produced in SAS GLIMMIX, though R presents more significant digits. The output for random effects is different in *R* from SAS or SPSS. The values for the intercept and standard deviation are in the logit scale, and the standard deviation is the square root of the variance of the random intercept estimate and not the standard error of the estimate. See http://www.ats.ucla.edu/stat/r/dae/melogit.htm for more information.

9.5.5 Two-Level Nested Logistic Regression Model Random Intercept and Slope with SAS

In these models, we believe the length of stay impacts other things during the previous visit and have an indirect varying effect for each patient. This varying effect is measured through the slope, for each patient. These slopes are members of a population of slopes with a mean and variance from a normal population. Thus, the intercept and the slope represent random effects, which are allowed to vary according to a normal distribution. Thus, the length of stay has a significant influence but does not affect all patients in the same way.

Two-Level Nested Logistic Regression Model Random Intercept and Slope with SAS GLIMMIX

SAS Program

```
GLIMMIX WITH RANDOM INTERCEPT AND RANDOM SLOPE
TITLE 'GLIMMIX WITH RANDOM COEFFICIENTS (RANDOM INTERCEPT AND
RANDOM SLOPE FOR LOS)';
PROC GLIMMIX DATA=MYDATA;
CLASS PNUM_R;
MODEL BIRADMIT (EVENT='1')=NDX NPR LOS DX101 T2 T3/DIST=BINARY
LINK=LOGIT DDFM=BW SOLUTION;
RANDOM INTERCEPT LOS/ SUBJECT =PNUM_R;
RUN;
```

Comment The slope now joins the set of random effects in the RANDOM statement through the LOS. We are assuming that each patient has their own slope as it pertains to LOS.

SAS Output

```
GLIMMIX WITH RANDOM COEFFICIENTS (RANDOM INTERCEPT AND RANDOM
SLOPE FOR LOS)
                      THE GLIMMIX PROCEDURE
                        MODEL INFORMATION
Dataset                        WORK.MYDATA
Response Variable               biRadmit
Response Distribution           Binary
Link Function                   Logit
Variance Function               Default
Variance Matrix Blocked By      PNUM_R
Estimation Technique            Residual PL
Degrees of Freedom Method       Between-Within
```

Comment This information addresses the properties used to fit the data.

```
                     CLASS LEVEL INFORMATION
Class     Levels    Values
PNUM_R    1625      127 560 746 750 1117 1395 1568 2076 2390 2413
3008 3123 3710 3970 3982 4236 4581 4873 5387 .........1370458
1370470 1371713
Number of Observations Read        4875
Number of Observations Used        4875
```

Comment This is a list of the clusters (patients) that provides the random effects.

```
                        RESPONSE PROFILE
Ordered                        Total
Value     biRadmit           Frequency
1         0                  2433
2         1                  2442
The GLIMMIX procedure is modeling the probability that
biRadmit='1'.
                           DIMENSIONS
G-side Cov. Parameters              2
```

Comment The G-side parameters are now two (intercept and slope). The matrix X still has seven parameters. With the random slope, there are now two parameters, slope and intercept.

```
Columns in X                         7
Columns in Z per Subject             2
Subjects (Blocks in V)            1625
Max Obs per Subject                  3
```

Comment There are seven columns in X representing Intercept, NDX, NPR, LOS, DX101, T_2 and T_3. There are two columns in Z, a column of ones and column of LOS.

```
                    OPTIMIZATION INFORMATION
Optimization technique        Newton-Raphson with ridging
```

Comment In fitting this model, we are using numerical techniques as there is no closed form. The optimization algorithm used is Newton-Raphson with ridging.

```
                         FIT STATISTICS
-2 Res Log Pseudo-Likelihood          20781.69
Generalized Chi-square                 4660.29
Gener. Chi-square / DF                    0.96
Comment: The ratio is expected to be one or close to one when the
model fits.
```

```
                COVARIANCE PARAMETER ESTIMATES
Standard
Cov Parm      Subject     Estimate        Error
Intercept     PNUM_R      0.1193          0.05646
LOS           PNUM_R      0.000886        0.000426
```

Comment Those estimates for the covariance can be used by computing the standardized values 0.1193/0.05646 = 2.113 (greater than 1.96) for the intercepts and 0.000886/0.000426 = 2.0798 (greater than 1.96) for the slopes to determine their significance. Thus, there are definite differences among the patients with regard to the length of stay over hospitalizations, meaning that each patient has a distinct intercept and slope.

Solutions for Fixed Effects

Effect	Estimate	Standard Error	DF	t Value	Pr > |t|
Intercept	-0.3563	0.1295	1624	-2.75	0.0060
NDX	0.06115	0.01582	3244	3.86	0.0001
NPR	-0.03214	0.01911	3244	-1.68	0.0928
LOS	0.03879	0.005984	3244	6.48	<.0001
DX101	-0.1086	0.09353	3244	-1.16	0.2456
T2	-0.3951	0.07203	3244	-5.49	<.0001
T3	-0.2455	0.07249	3244	-3.39	0.0007

Comment The fitted logistic regression model is $\log\left(\hat{P}_{y=1} | \hat{P}_{y=0}\right) = -0.356 + 0.061\text{NDX} - 0.032\text{NPR} + 0.039\text{LOS} - 0.108\text{DX101} - 0.395\text{T}_2 - 0.245\text{T}_3$ ·
The covariates, NDX, LOS, T_2 and T_3,are significant. The link is logit.

Comment These tests are for the fixed effects and are based on F-test. Since $=t^2$, the results are the same as the t-test in the earlier frame. Only NDX and LOS are significant.

Two-Level Nested Logistic Regression Model Random Intercept and Slope with SAS NLMIXED

SAS PROGRAM NLMIXED

```
WITH RANDOM INTERCEPT AND RANDOM SLOPE FOR LOS
PROC NLMIXED DATA=MYDATA;
PARMS b0=-0.3675 b1=0.0648 b2=-0.0306 b3=0.0344 b4=-0.1143
b5=-0.3876 b6=-0.2412 S2U=1  S2LOS=1 ;
ETA=U+b0+b1*NDX+b2*NPR+b3*LOS+b4*DX101+b5*T2+b6*T3+RB1*LOS;
EXPETA=EXP(ETA);
P=(EXPETA/(1+EXPETA));
MODEL BIRADMIT ~ BINARY (P);
RANDOM U RB1 ~ NORMAL ([0, 0], [S2U, 0, S2LOS]) SUBJECT=PNUM_R;
RUN;
```

Comment The slope RB1 (random slope) is now a random effect in the model. It is entered through the use of the RANDOM statement. So, both intercept (U) with mean zero and variance S_{2u} with the slope (RB1) mean zero and variance S_{2u} are random such that $\begin{pmatrix} Intercept \\ Slope \end{pmatrix} \sim \mathcal{N}\begin{pmatrix} S_{2u} & 0 \\ 0 & S_{2LOS} \end{pmatrix}$.

SAS Output

```
NLMIXED: RANDOM COEFFICIENTS (RANDOM INTERCEPT AND RANDOM SLOPE)


                        PARAMETER ESTIMATES
                  Standard
Parameter Estimate  Error  DF  t Value Pr > |t|  Alpha Lower
Upper   Gradient
b0  -0.369  0.134  1623  -2.74  0.006  0.05  -0.633 -0.1048 0.004
b1   0.059  0.0167 1623   3.52  0.0004 0.05   0.026  0.092 0.0323
b2  -0.035  0.020  1623  -1.76  0.078  0.05  -0.07483
0.004015 0.037
b3   0.050  0.008  1623   6.06  <.0001 0.05   0.03369
0.06593 0.091
b4  -0.099  0.098  1623  -1.01  0.312  0.05  -0.292 0.093  -0.005
b5  -0.420  0.075  1623  -5.63  <.0001 0.05  -0.5672 -0.274 0.003
b6  -0.258  0.075  1623  -3.45  0.001  0.05  -0.4060 -0.1117 0.001
S2U  0.175  0.083  1623   2.12  0.035  0.05   0.0128 0.337  0.001
S2LOS 0.003 0.001  1623   1.99  0.047  0.05   0.00034
0.005 -0.219
```

Comment The fitted logistic regression model is $\log\left(\hat{P}_{y=1}|\hat{P}_{y=0}\right) = -0.356 + 0.061\text{NDX} - 0.032\text{NPR} + 0.039\text{LOS} - 0.108\text{DX}101 - 0.395\text{T}_2 - 0.245\text{T}_3$ · The covariates, NDX, LOS, T_2 and T_3,are significant. The link is logit. We got similar results with PROC GLIMMIX and NLMIXED.

9.5.6 Two-Level Nested Logistic Regression Model Random Intercept and Slope with SPSS

SPSS Program

We use SPSS to fit the two-level nested logistic regression model with random intercept and random slope.

```
GENLINMIXED
  /DATA_STRUCTURE SUBJECTS=PNUM_R
  /FIELDS TARGET=biRadmit TRIALS=NONE OFFSET=NONE
  /TARGET_OPTIONS DISTRIBUTION=BINOMIAL LINK=LOGIT
  /FIXED EFFECTS=NDX NPR LOS DX101 T2 T3 USE_INTERCEPT=TRUE
  /RANDOM EFFECTS=LOS USE_INTERCEPT=TRUE SUBJECTS=PNUM_R
COVARIANCE_TYPE=VARIANCE_COMPONENTS
  /BUILD_OPTIONS TARGET_CATEGORY_ORDER=ASCENDING INPUTS_CATEGORY_
ORDER=ASCENDING MAX_ITERATIONS=100 CONFIDENCE_LEVEL=95 DF_
METHOD=RESIDUAL COVB=MODEL
  /EMMEANS_OPTIONS SCALE=ORIGINAL PADJUST=LSD.
```

Comment Similar to the logistic regression model with random intercept and that output, SPSS performs a significance test automatically for both the random intercept and slope. Note the fewer significant digits that may limit our ability to report values precisely (particularly a standard error for the length of stay (LOS) of zero).

Comment Here are the fixed effects parameter estimates with similar notes to the random intercept only model, highlighting differences in displaying significant digits, the reference category used, and the signs of certain estimates. Similar interpretations can be made using SPSS, though care must be taken to ensure the correct reference category is being discussed.

Model 2: Logistic Regression with Random Intercept/Random Slope for LOS

SPSS Output

Fixed Coefficients
Target: biRadmit
Reference category: 0

Model term	Coefficient	Std. error	t	Sig.	Lower	Upper
Intercept	−0.356	0.129	−2.751	0.006	−0.610	−0.102
NDX	0.061	0.016	3.865	0.000	0.030	0.092
NPR	−0.032	0.019	−1.681	0.093	−0.070	0.005
LOS	0.039	0.006	6.482	0.000	0.027	0.051
DX101	−0.109	0.094	−1.161	0.246	−0.292	0.075
T2 = 1	−0.395	0.072	−5.485	0.000	−0.536	−0.254
T3 = 1	−0.246	0.072	−3.327	0.001	−0.388	−0.103

Comment: The fitted logistic regression model is $\log\left(\hat{P}_{y=1} \mid \hat{P}_{y=0}\right) =$

$$-0.356 + 0.061\text{NDX} - 0.032\text{NPR} + 0.039\text{LOS} - 0.109\text{DX101} - 0.395\text{T}_2 - 0.246\text{T}_3$$

. The covariates, NDX, LOS, T_2 and T_3,are significant. The link is logit
Probability distribution: Binomial
Link function: Logit
[a]This coefficient is set to zero because it is redundant

Covariance Parameters
Target: biRadmit

Covariance parameters	Residual effect	0
	Random effects	2
Design matrix columns	Fixed effects	9
	Random effects	2[a]
Common subjects		1625

Comment: Common subjects are based on the subject specifications for the residual and random effects and are used to chunk the data for better performance

[a]This is the number of columns per common subject

Random effect	Estimate	Std. error	Z	Sig.	95% confidence interval	
					Lower	Upper
Var(intercept)	0.119	0.056	2.113	0.035	0.047	0.302
Var(LOS)	0.001	0.000	2.081	0.037	0.000	0.002

Covariance structure: Variance components
Subject specification: PNUM_R

Comment The estimate of variance of the random effects is 0.119 with a 95% confidence interval of (0.047, 0.302). This suggests that the variance is significantly different from zero. Thus, the random effects are present. An estimate of the variance of the slope is 0.001 with a 95% confidence interval of (0.000, 0.002) and p-value of 0.037. Thus, the patients have different rates of change when length of stay is considered.

9.5.7 *Two-Level Nested Logistic Regression Model Random Intercept and Slope with STATA*

STATA

```
. melogit biRadmit NDX NPR LOS DX101 T2 T3 || PNUM_R: LOS
```

Fitting fixed effects model:

```
Iteration 2:  Log likelihood = -3316.3284
Mixed-effects logistic regression        Number of obs     =     4,875
Group variable: PNUM_R                   Number of groups =     1,625
Obs per group:
min =        3
avg =        3.0
max =        3
Integration method: mvaghermite          Integration pts.  =         7
Wald chi2(6)         =       107.76
Log likelihood = -3302.3832              Prob > chi2       =    0.0000
biRadmit  Coefficient  Std. err.     z     P>z     [95% conf. interval]
NDX     .0589919    .0167419     3.52   0.000    .0261784    .0918054
NPR   -.0357382    .0200984    -1.78   0.075   -.0751303    .003654
LOS     .049875     .0082371     6.05   0.000    .0337306    .0660194
DX101 -.0947255    .0979593    -0.97   0.334   -.2867222    .0972712
T2    -.4204694    .0747545    -5.62   0.000   -.5669856   -.2739533
T3    -.2585956    .0750296    -3.45   0.001   -.4056509   -.1115403
_cons -.3696249    .1344916    -2.75   0.006   -.6332235   -.1060262
PNUM_R
var(LOS)    .0025381    .0013113              .000922     .0069869
var(_cons) .173659     .0829037              .0681302     .4426448
LR test vs. logistic model: chi2(2) = 27.89     Prob > chi2 = 0.0000
```

Note: LR test is conservative and provided only for reference.

9.6 Conclusions

In Chap. 6, we presented the GEE logistic regression model as a means of addressing correlated data. We pointed out that this method of analyzing correlated data was done through the random component. In this chapter, we presented a generalized linear mixed model as another approach to analyzing correlated data. This method of analysis of correlated data was done through the systematic component. We reiterate that these two methods of analysis are not necessarily answering the same question. One model presents the probability of rehospitalization and the other model tells us about the probability of rehospitalization for a particular patient. We found that the probability of a patient being rehospitalized in 30 days depends on the length of stay and the number of prescriptions. We found that the assumption of independence realizes smaller standard errors as opposed to correlated data. It is evident that the marginal model (Chap. 6) provides results that are different than those from the subject-specific model, unless the random effects are not significant. Thus, it is relevant to ask the question, *how do they compare?* While the GEE model provides a simple alternative for correlated clustered data, is computationally simple, and robust against misspecification of correlation structures, it is not necessarily efficient. As such, the interpretations of the fixed effect coefficient in a GEE model are usually different than those in the generalized linear mixed model. The GEE model has a covariance structure mainly due to the random component referred to as the R-side, while the generalized linear mixed model has a covariance structure due to the random and systematic components. This results in two sides to the covariance structure: the R- and G-side. More importantly, GEE fits marginal models, while PROC GLIMMIX fits subject-specific models.

9.7 Related Examples

9.7.1 Multicenter Randomized Controlled Data (Beitler & Landis, 1985)

A similar set of data that may necessitate this type of analysis is multicenter randomized controlled data (Beitler & Landis, 1985; Wolfinger, 1999). Data are collected in a multicenter randomized controlled clinical trial conducted in eight different clinics. The primary purpose of the study is to assess the effect of a topical cream treatment on curing nonspecific infections, as compared to a placebo. In each of the eight clinics, the numbers of treated persons and successfully cured persons are recorded for both the treatment and placebo groups. This is an example of patients nested within clinics. The data as presented by Kuss: How to Use SAS for Logistic Regression with Correlated Data, SUGI 2002, Orlando.

```
DATA INFECTION;
INPUT CLINIC TREATMENT X N;
DATALINES;
1  1  11  36
1  0  10  37
...
8 1 4 6
8 0 6 7
RUN;
```

One may be interested in certain questions such as:

1. Does the treatment impact the cure?
2. Is there an impact of the clinic on the cure?
3. What are the results if we had treatment and clinic simultaneously on cure with clinic as a fixed effect?
4. What are the results if we had treatment and clinic simultaneously on cure with clinic as a random effect?

References

Allison, P. D. (1999). *Logistic regression using the SAS system*. SAS Institute.

Beitler, P. J., & Landis, J. R. (1985). A mixed-effects model for categorical data. *Biometrics, 41*, 991–1000.

Blackwelder, W. C., Armitage, P., & Colton, T. (1998). *Encyclopedia of statistics*. Wiley.

Breslow, N. E., & Clayton, D. G. (1993). Approximate inference in generalized linear mixed models. *Journal of the American Statistical Association, 88*(421), 9–25.

Dean, C. B., & Nielsen, J. D. (2007). Generalized linear mixed models: A review and some extensions. *Lifetime Data Analysis, 13*(4), 497–512.

Fernée, C., & Trimmis, K. (2021). Detecting variability: A study on the application of Bayesian multilevel modelling to archaeological data. Evidence from the Neolithic Adriatic and the Bronze Age Aegean. *Journal of Archaeological Science, 128*. https://doi.org/10.1016/j.jas.2021.105346

Goldstein, H. (2003). *Multilevel statistical models* (3rd ed.). Edward Arnold.

Have, T. R., Kunselman, A. R., & Tran, L. (1999). A comparison of mixed effects logistic regression models for binary response data with two nested levels of clustering. *Statistics in Medicine, 18*, 947–960.

Hox, J. J. (2002). *Multilevel analysis: Techniques and applications*. Lawrence Erlbaum Associates.

Hox, J. J., & Maas, C. J. (2002). *Sample sizes for multilevel modeling* (pp. 1–19). Utrecht University. Retrieved from: igitur-archive.library.uu.nl

Hu, F. B., Goldberg, J., Hedeker, D., Flay, B. R., & Pentz, M. A. (1998). Comparison of population-averaged and subject-specific approaches for analyzing repeated binary outcomes. *American Journal of Epidemiology, 147*(7), 694–703.

Larsen, K., Petersen, J. H., Budtz-Jorgensen, E., & Endahl, L. (2000). Interpreting parameters in the logistic regression model with random effects. *Biometrics, 56*, 909–914.

Longford, N. T. (1993). *Random coefficient models*. Clarendon Press.

McCulloch, C. E. (2003, January). Generalized linear mixed models. In *NSF-CBMS regional conference series in probability and statistics* (pp. i–84). Institute of Mathematical Statistics and the American Statistical Association.

Murray, D. M., Varnell, S. P., & Blitstein, J. L. (2004). Design and analysis of group-randomized trials: A review of recent methodological developments. *Journal Information, 94*(3).

Schabenberger, O. (2005). Introducing the GLIMMIX procedure for generalized linear mixed models. *SUGI 30 Proceedings*, 196-30.

Wolfinger, R. (1993). Covariance structure selection in general mixed models. *Communications in Statistics-Simulation and Computation, 22*(4), 1079–1106.

Wolfinger, R. D. (1999). *Fitting nonlinear mixed models with the new NLMIXED procedure*. Proceedings of the 24th Annual SAS Users Group.

Chapter 10
Hierarchical Logistic Regression Models

10.1 Motivation

10.1.1 Description of Case Study

In surveys of discharged patients from hospitals, it is common for administrators to obtain a measure of the patient's overall experience at the hospital upon discharge. Therefore, identifying factors that contribute to making patients' stays better is of the utmost importance. As such, hospital administrators are interested in knowing the responses from patients who are hospitalized for different reasons with different procedures and with a specific number of prescriptions as well as their medical histories, among other things. For planning purposes, they may wish to identify any significant characteristics of the doctors that contributes to the patients' satisfaction levels.

In this chapter, we are going to look at a set of questions about overall hospital stay experience designed for cancer patients in remission. We will model cancer remission as it pertains to hospital differentials in terms of patients' characteristics, doctor's experience, and size of the hospital.

Data simulated with hospitals, doctors, and patients (HDP) are analyzed in this chapter. This dataset consists of a three-level, hierarchical structure with patients nested within doctors and doctors nested within hospitals. We used the simulated data to show a variety of analytical techniques as they pertain to fitting logistic regression models to hierarchical data. The simulated data are meant to be a large study of lung cancer outcomes across multiple doctors and hospitals (www.ats.ucla.edu/stat/r/pages/mesimulation.htm).

J. R. Wilson et al., *Modeling Binary Correlated Responses*, ICSA Book Series in Statistics, https://doi.org/10.1007/978-3-031-62427-8_10

10.1.2 Study Hypotheses

The hierarchical logistic regression models incorporate the different sources of variations. At each level of the hierarchy, we use random effects and other appropriate fixed effects. This chapter demonstrates the fit of hierarchical logistic regression models with random intercepts and random intercepts and random slopes to the multilevel data. If we were to use the standard binomial logistic regression model to analyze such hierarchical data, we would be ignoring several sources of variation. Instead, we use a hierarchical model to identify factors such as testing how patients' characteristics, doctors' experience, and hospitals' factors contribute to the remission.

10.2 Definitions and Notations

Nested, hierarchical, and multilevel are different terms essentially representing the same concept.

Nested design is a design in which every level of a given factor appears within only a single level of any other factor.

Hierarchical, as the word implies, is a level of hierarchy where a classification is arranged in levels, usually in order of rank. Hierarchical data consist of units grouped at different levels.

Multilevel modeling allows modeling to distinguish multiple levels of information in a model. Coefficients can be fixed or random and, as such, at one level can be presented on the input and at the next level can be output.

Complete separation occurs when the response variable separates a predictor variable or a combination of predictor variables completely. You do not need the predictors to tell you of the next output value. See Table 10.1.

In this example, the response is zero when covariate X is less than 5 and 1 when the covariate X is more than 4. So, covariate X predicts the response perfectly. This is realized without having to do any kind of estimation. Thus mathematically, the maximum likelihood estimate for the X coefficient does not exist.

Table 10.1 Demonstration of separation

Response C	Covariate X	Covariate W	Response S	Covariate X2	Covariate W2
0	1	0	0	1	0
0	2	1	0	2	1
0	3	0	0	3	0
0	4	1	0	4	1
1	5	0	1	4	0
1	6	0	1	6	0
1	7	1	1	7	1

Quasi-separation in a logistic regression occurs when the outcome variable separates a predictor variable or a combination of predictor variables to certain degree. The response S separates the covariate X2 except for values of X2 = 4. Thus, the covariate predicts perfectly when X2 is less than 4 or greater than 4. The maximum likelihood estimate for the coefficient of X2 does not exist (http://www.ats.ucla.edu/stat/mult_pkg/faq/general/complete_separation_logit_models.htm).

10.3 Exploratory Analyses

It is common to be presented with data that have hierarchical or nested clustered structures. Examples include patients within a hospital, hospitals within counties, students within a class, and classes within a school (all at two-level structures). Examples of three-level structures would be factories within an industry within states or families within a neighborhood within cities (all three levels). In such cases, there is variability between the clusters as well as variability between the units, which are nested within the clusters. Modeling hierarchical data should include the variability at each level of the hierarchy and thus allow for the cluster effects at different levels to be analyzed within the models (Shahian et al., 2001). We are interested in how one can incorporate the information from different levels into a model, thereby presenting a subject-specific logistic regression model.

In this chapter, we concentrate on fitting logistic regression models to these kinds of nested data at three levels and higher. In Fig. 10.1, we have patients nested within doctors and doctors nested within hospitals, making it a three-level nested design. We wish to fit of a logistic regression model to reflect the differences between doctors and between hospitals.

If we were to use the standard logistic regression model to these data with remission event = 1 and age, length of stay, (as patient's information), and experience (as the doctor's information) as covariates, we will receive the following results:

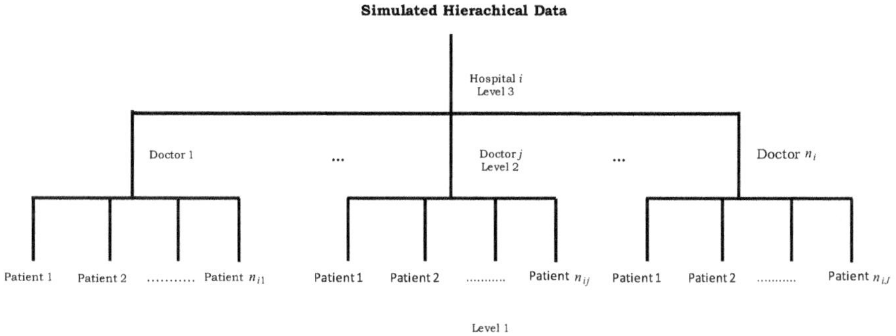

Fig. 10.1 Nested structure of the hospital, doctor, and patient

Criterion	Intercept Only	Intercept and Covariates
AIC	10354.637	10038.505
SC	10361.688	10066.708
-2 Log L	10352.637	10030.505

TESTING GLOBAL NULL HYPOTHESIS: BETA=0

Test	Chi-Square	DF	Pr > ChiSq
Likelihood Ratio	322.1325	3	<.0001
Score	316.5248	3	<.0001
Wald	304.8871	3	<.0001

Analysis of Maximum Likelihood Estimates

Parameter	DF	Estimate	Standard Error	Wald Chi-Square	Pr > ChiSq
Intercept	1	-0.2882	0.2254	1.6348	0.2010
Age	1	-0.0213	0.00434	23.9521	<.0001
Length of Stay	1	-0.1842	0.0260	50.1282	<.0001
Experience	1	0.0838	0.00605	192.0264	<.0001

Odds Ratio Estimates

Effect	Point Estimate	95% Wald Confidence Limits	
Age	0.979	0.971	0.987
Length of Stay	0.832	0.790	0.875
Experience	1.087	1.075	1.100

It appears that age, length of stay, and the doctor's experience have significant impact on cancer remission. However, this analysis ignores the fact that age and length of stay are measured on patients who are nested within doctors and experience is measured on the doctors who are nested within the hospitals.

10.4 Statistical Model

It is common in fields such as public health, education, demography, and sociology to encounter data structures where the information is collected based on a hierarchy. An appropriate approach to analyze such data is, therefore, to include the nested sources of variability coming from the different levels of the hierarchy. The different levels provide variability that must be accounted for. The total variability consists of several components. At each level, there is intraclass correlation as there are units within clusters and between units at different levels. This type of hierarchy results in correlated data. As a result of the correlation at each level inherent from these hierarchical structures, the standard logistic regression model is inappropriate (Rasbash et al., 2012).

10.4.1 Multilevel Modeling Approaches with Binary Outcomes

Binary outcomes are very common in healthcare research, for example, one may refer to the patient who has improved or recovered after discharge from the hospital or not. For healthcare and other types of research, a logistic regression model is one of the preferred methods of modeling data when the outcome variable is binary. In its standard form, it is a member of a class of generalized linear models specific to the binomial random component. As is customary in regression analysis, it makes use of several predictor variables that may be either numerical or categorical. However, a standard logistic regression model assumes that the observations obtained from each unit are independent. If we were to fit a standard logistic regression to nested data, the assumption of independent observations is seriously violated. This violation could lead to an underestimation of the standard errors and as such declare significance when in fact it is not.

One common approach when analyzing nested data is, therefore, to use multilevel models approaches while incorporating nested sources of variability at each level. One approach for multilevel linear modeling but applied to dyadic data analysis with continuous outcomes is seen (Raudenbush, 1992). That work was extended with two-level approaches with binary outcomes (McMahon et al., 2006).

In this chapter, we analyze three-level nested data, but it is possible to analyze data higher level data. The key with higher level lies with the use random effect at each level. We make use of two models each with two random effects at level 2 and level 3 with random intercept only and with random intercept and random slopes. For analysis of multilevel data, random effects are added into the model to account for unobservable effects that are known to exist but are not measured. Here, we will consider two models at three levels. One is a model with random effects at level 2 and level 3. The other models the data with random intercepts and random slopes at levels 2 and 3.

10.4.2 Potential Problems

We found that convergence of parameter estimates is sometimes difficult to achieve, especially when fitting models with random slopes and higher levels of nesting. Some researchers have found that convergence problems may occur if the outcome is skewed for certain clusters or if there is quasi separation or complete separation. Such phenomena destroy the variability within clusters which is essential to the solutions. In addition, we found that including too many random effects may not be computationally possible (Schabenberger, 2005).

We also found what other researchers did. That for hierarchal logistic models for nested binary data, it is often not feasible to estimate random effects for both intercepts and slopes at the same time in a model. Also, Newsom (2002) showed that we can have models with too many parameters to be estimated given the number of covariance elements included. Others found that such models can lead to severe convergence problems, limiting the modeling. Before fitting these conditional models, McMahon et al. (2006) suggested that one should determine whether there is significant cluster interdependence to justify the use of multilevel modeling. For the simulated data, we fit random slopes at different levels without random intercepts. The fit of these models is performed through SAS with PROC NLMIXED as well as SPSS and R. One researcher claimed that only one random statement is supported in PROC NLMIXED so that nonlinear mixed models cannot be assessed at more than two levels (Maas & Hox, 2004). However, Hedeker et al. (2008, 2012) showed how more than one random statement can be used for continuous data in PROC NLMIXED with more than two levels. We adopted some of their techniques and applied them to the analysis of binary data when using PROC NLMIXED in SAS. We fit models with random effects using SAS.

10.4.3 Three-Level Logistic Regression Models with Multiple Random Intercepts

In the analysis of multilevel data, each level provides a component of variance that measures intraclass correlation. Consider a hierarchical model at three levels for the kth patient seeing the jth doctor in the ith hospital. The patients are at the lower level (level 1) and are nested within doctors (level 2), which are nested within hospitals at the next level (level 3). We consider the hospital as the primary unit, doctors as the secondary unit, and patients as the observational unit. These clusters are treated as random effects. We make use of random effects as we believe there are some nonmeasurable benefits based on the doctor and also based on the hospital. Some effects may be positive, and some effects may be negative, but overall, we assume their average is zero.

At level 1, we take responses from different patients noting their age (age) and length of stay (LOS). Then, the outcomes are modeled through a logistic regression model

$$\log\left[\frac{p_{ijk}}{1-p_{ijk}}\right] = \gamma_{oij} + \gamma_{1ij}\text{Age}_{ijk} + \gamma_{2ij}\text{Los}_{ijk} \tag{10.1}$$

where γ_{oij} is the intercept, γ_{1ij} is the coefficient associated with the predictor Age_{ijk}, and γ_{2ij} is the coefficient associated with the predictor Los_{ijk} (length of stay) for $k = 1,2, \ldots, n_{ij}$ patients; $j = 1, 2, \ldots, n_i$ doctors and $i = 1, \ldots, n$; hospitals. Each doctor has a separate logistic model. If we allow the effects of age and LOS on the outcome to be the same for each doctor but allow the intercept to be different than on the logit scale, we have parallel planes for their predictive model. The γ_{oij} intercept represents those differential effects among doctors.

At level 2, we assume that the intercept γ_{oij} (which allows a different intercept for doctors within hospitals) depends on the unobserved factors specific to the ith hospital, the covariates given as associated with the doctors of the ith hospital, and a random effect u_{oij} associated with doctor j within hospital i. Thus,

$$\gamma_{oij} = \gamma_{oi} + \gamma_{1i}\text{Experience}_{ij} + u_{oij} \tag{10.2}$$

where Experience_{ij} is the experience for doctor j of the ith hospital. Similarly, hospital administration policies may have different effects on doctors. At level 3, the model assumes that differential hospital policies depend on the overall fixed intercept β_0 and the random effect u_{oi} associated with the intercept for hospital i. Thus,

$$\gamma_{oi} = \beta_0 + u_{oi}. \tag{10.3}$$

By successive substitution into the expression for γ_{oi} in (10.3) into (10.2) and then by substituting the resulting expression for γ_{oij}into (10.1), we obtain

$$\log\left[\frac{p_{ijk}}{1-p_{ijk}}\right] = \beta_0 + \gamma_{1i}\text{Experience}_{ij} + \gamma_{1ij}\text{Age}_{ijk} + \gamma_{2ij}\text{Los}_{ijk} + u_{oi} + u_{oij} \tag{10.4}$$

The combination of random and fixed terms results in a generalized linear mixed model with two random effects, hospitals denoted by $u_{oi} \sim \mathcal{N}\left(0,\sigma^2_{u_i}\right)$ and doctors denoted by $u_{oij} \sim \mathcal{N}\left(0,\sigma^2_{u_{ij}}\right)$ with covariance $\sigma_{u_{oi},\,u_{oij}}$. From (10.4), the model consists of all overall mean plus experience of doctors plus age of patient and length of stay plus effects due to hospitals and effects due to doctors for each individual. Hence, we have a subject-specific model.

10.4.4 Three-Level Logistic Regression Models with Random Intercepts and Random Slopes

Consider the three-level random intercept and random slope model consisting of a logistic regression model at level 1,

$$\log\left[\frac{p_{ijk}}{1-p_{ijk}}\right] = \gamma_{oij} + \gamma_{1ij}\text{Age}_{ijk} + \gamma_{2ij}\text{Los}_{ijk} \tag{10.5}$$

where both γ_{oij} and γ_{2ij} are random, for k = 1,2, …, n_{ij}; j = 1, 2, …, n_i; and i = 1, …, n. So, each doctor has a different intercept and the rates of change with respect to age and for length of stay are not the same for all the doctors. However, there are some unobserved effects related to LOS that impact remission. There are factors associated with LOS and the doctors' impacts on patients vary as LOS varies. The intercept represents a group of unidentifiable factors that impact the overall effect of the doctor on the patient's success, while the slope represents the differential impact that the particular variable (LOS) has that results in differences among patients.

So, at level 2, γ_{oij} and γ_{2ij} are treated as response variables within the model,

$$\gamma_{oij} = \gamma_{oi} + \gamma_{1i}\text{Experience}_{ij} + u_{oij} \tag{10.6}$$

$$\gamma_{2ij} = \gamma_{2i} + u_{2ij} \tag{10.7}$$

where γ_{oi} and γ_{2i} are random effects. Equation (10.6) assumes the intercept γ_{oij} for doctors nested within hospital j, the unobserved intercept specific to the ith hospital, the effects associated with the doctor's experience in the hospital, and a random term u_{oij} associated with doctor j within hospital i. The slope γ_{2ij} depends on the overall slope γ_{2i} for hospital i and a random term u_{2ij}.

$$\gamma_{oi} = \beta_{00} + u_{oi} \tag{10.8}$$

$$\gamma_{2i} = \beta_{22} + u_{2i} \tag{10.9}$$

At level 3, the model shows that the hospitals vary based on random effects and that the intercept depends on the overall fixed intercept β_{00} and the random term u_{oi} associated with the hospital *i,* while the hospital slope γ_{2i} depends on the overall fixed slope β_{22} and the random effect u_{2i} associated with the slope for hospital i. By substituting the expression for γ_{oi} and γ_{2i} into (10.7) and (10.8) and then substituting the resulting expression for γ_{oij} and γ_{2ij}into (10.9), we obtained

$$\log\left[\frac{p_{ijk}}{1-p_{ijk}}\right] = \beta_{00} + \gamma_{1ij}\text{Age}_{ijk} + \gamma_{1i}\text{Experience}_{ij} + u_{oi} + u_{oij} + \left(\beta_{22} + u_{2i} + u_{2ij}\right)\text{Los}_{ijk}. \tag{10.10}$$

Thus, we have a generalized linear mixed model with random effects u_{oi}, u_{oij}, γ_{1i} and γ_{1ij}. Therefore, Los_{ijk} is associated with both a fixed and random part. We take advantage of this regrouping of terms to incorporate the random effects and their variance-covariance matrix, so that u_{oi}, u_{oij}, γ_{1i}, and γ_{1ij} are jointly distributed normally with a mean of zero and a covariance matrix reflecting the relationships between the random effects.

10.4.5 Nested Higher Level Logistic Regression Models

For higher than three-level nested, we can easily present the model, though executing the necessary computations must be tedious. Imagine if we had the data with another level, hospitals nested within cities (level 4 denoted by *h*). Cities may have their own way of monitoring healthcare within their jurisdiction. We also believed that the number of beds within the hospital is a necessary variable. For such we will have kth patient nested within the jth doctor that is nested within i^{th} hospital, which is nested into the hth city. Then, the model is as follows:

$$\log\left[\frac{p_{hijk}}{1-p_{hijk}}\right] = \beta_{00} + \gamma_{1hij}\text{Age}_{hijk} + \gamma_{1hi}\text{Experience}_{hij} + \gamma_{1h}\text{Bed}_{hi} + u_{oh} + u_{ohi} + u_{ohij} + \left(\beta_{22} + u_{2hi} + u_{2hij}\right)\text{Los}_{hijk} \tag{10.11}$$

10.4.6 Cluster Sizes and Number of Clusters

Regardless of the number of clusters, Austin (2010) found that for all statistical software procedures, the estimation of variance components tended to be poor when there are only five subjects per cluster. The number of clusters on the mean number of quadrature points is negligible. However, when the random effects are large, Rodriquez and Goldman (1995) found substantial decreases in the estimation of fixed effects and/or variance components. They also found that there was bias in the estimation when the number of subjects per cluster was small.

10.4.7 Parameter Estimations

The joint distribution of conditional distribution of the responses and the distribution of the random effects provides a joint likelihood not necessarily readily written in closed form. However, we still need to estimate the regression coefficients and the random components. In so doing, it is imperative for us to use some form of approximations. Sometimes researchers have used the quasi-likelihood approach through a Taylor series expansion to approximate the joint likelihood. The approximate likelihood is maximized to produce maximized quasi-likelihood estimates.

The disadvantage that many have pointed out with this approach is the bias involved with quasi-likelihoods (Wedderburn, 1974). Others researchers have resorted to numerical integration approximation of the true likelihood. These integrals are split up into quadratures. The more quadratures, the more accurate is the result. More integration points will increase the number of computations and thus impede the speed of convergence, although it increases the accuracy. Each added random component increases the integral dimension. A random intercept is one dimension (one added parameter), a random slope is two dimensions. Our experience is that the three-level nested models with random intercepts and slopes often create problems regarding convergence. There were analyses where we have to try certain options to get convergence.

10.5 Analysis of Data

10.5.1 Modeling Random Intercepts for Levels 2 and 3

We fitted a logistic regression model (10.4) with random effects for doctors and hospitals, covariates age, and length of stay at the patient level and experience at the doctor level. We used SAS R and STATA to fit these models.

10.5.2 Modeling Random Intercepts for Levels 2 and 3

Modeling Random Intercepts for Levels 2 and 3 Using SAS

We use PROC NLMIXED with the Qpoints option and also with the ABSFCONV option. We find that making use of these options sometimes facilitated convergence. We demonstrate the use of the Qpoints and then we look at the ABSFCONV.

SAS Program

```
/* Model with random effects of u0 (hospital) and u01 (doctors)*/
proc nlmixed data= HDPDATA  Qpoints= 80;
parms b0=3.4462 b1=0.01128 b2=-0.04626 b4=0.0925 s11=1.2
s22=1 c12=-1;
xb = b0 + u0 +u01+ b1*Age+b2*LengthofStay+b4*Experience;
p = exp(xb)/(1+exp(xb));
model remission ~ binary(p);
random u0 u01~ normal([0, 0],[s11,c12, s22]) subject=DID;
run;
```

Comment Option *Qpoints* helps to get convergence. *Parms* is used to provide these starting values. We recommend getting those values from the standard logistic regression for the coefficients and being conservative by choosing values for the variance component as one and that should suffice. The random term provides (Hedeker et al., 2012)

$$\begin{pmatrix} u_0 \\ u_1 \end{pmatrix} \sim \begin{pmatrix} 0 \\ 0 \end{pmatrix}, \begin{pmatrix} s_{11} & c_{12} \\ c_{21} & s_{22} \end{pmatrix}$$

s_{11} refers to the variance for hospitals as random effects, and s_{22} refers to the variance for doctors as random effects. Subject = DID represents the doctors ID, the first level of clustering. Patients are nested within doctors.

SAS Output

The NLMIXED **Procedure**

Specifications	
Dataset	WORK.HDPDATA
Dependent variable	Remission
Distribution for dependent variable	Binary
Random effects	u_0 u_1
Distribution for random effects	Normal
Subject variable	DID
Optimization technique	Dual quasi-Newton
Integration method	Adaptive Gaussian quadrature

Comment u_0 and u_1 are the random effects; normal specifies the distribution of the random effects; DID is the doctor's identity number; dual Quasi-Newton and adaptive Gaussian quadrature identify the method used to integrate the joint likelihood.

Dimensions	
Observations used	8525
Observations not used	0
Total observations	8525
Subjects	407
Max Obs per subject	40
Parameters	7
Quadrature points	80

Comment There were 8525 patients and 407 doctors, with a max number of patients as 40 with 7 parameters. We used as many as 80 quadrature points to get convergence.

Parameters							
b0	**b1**	**b2**	**b4**	**s11**	**s22**	**c12**	**NegLogLike**
3.4462	0.01128	−0.04626	0.0925	1.2	1	−1	21,352.1772

Comment These are the starting values as needed. One can obtain these from the standard logistic regression model. The covariance parameters can start with one as an initial value.

Iteration history					
Iter	**Calls**	**NegLogLike**	**Diff**	**MaxGrad**	**Slope**
1	6	4884.74367	16467.43	39063.7	−7.926E8
17	36	3837.72835	0.000113	1.804009	−0.00018
18	38	3837.72834	0.000011	0.184286	−8.6E-6

NOTE: GCONV convergence criterion satisfied

Comment Convergence was achieved. Note the difference in negative log likelihood (NegLogLike) is very small (iteration 17 to iteration 18). Also, the slope is almost zero at the stopping point.

Fit statistics	
−2 log-likelihood	7675.5
AIC (smaller is better)	7689.5
AICC (smaller is better)	7689.5
BIC (smaller is better)	7717.5

Comment −2 Log-likelihood = 7675.5 = 2*3837.72834 (from the last line of the iterations). These are fit statistic values. Since there are no *p*-values attached, it does not tell about the fit and its significance.

Parameter estimates									
Parameter	**Estimate**	**Standard error**	**DF**	**t value**	**Pr > |t|**	**Alpha**	**Lower**	**Upper**	**Gradient**
b0	−0.450	0.544	405	−0.83	0.4092	0.05	−1.520	0.621	0.004
b1(Age)	−0.033	0.0064	405	−5.89	<0.0001	0.05	−0.043	−0.022	0.184
b2(Los)	−0.260	0.033	405	−7.89	<0.0001	0.05	−0.325	−0.195	0.054
b4(Experience)	0.118	0.027	405	4.46	<0.0001	0.05	0.067	0.170	0.133
s11	1.795	0.064	405	27.96	<0.0001	0.05	1.669	1.921	0.001
s22	1.595	0.064	405	24.84	<0.0001	0.05	1.469	1.721	0.001
c12	0.190	0.128	405	1.48	0.1391	0.05	−0.062	0.443	0.001

Comment The logistic regression model is

$$\log\left(\frac{\hat{P}_{y=1|\text{random effect}}}{\hat{P}_{y=0}\,|\text{random effect}}\right) = -0.450 - 0.033\text{Age} - 0.260\text{Los} + 0.118\text{Experience}$$

The variance components s11 and s22 are significant (<0.0001) and the covariance c12 is not significant (0.1391). Thus, the variability among doctors ($\widehat{\sigma_{11}^2}$ 1.795) is significant (<0.0001), and the variability among hospitals ($\widehat{\sigma_{22}^2} = 1.595$) is significant (<0.0001). It makes good sense to include these random effects. Seeing certain doctors or having stayed at certain hospitals has an impact on patient's remission.

An Alternative SAS Program Making Use of Option ABSFCONV

```
proc nlmixed data= HDPDATA  ABSFCONV= 0.4;
parms b0=3.4462 b1=0.01128 b2=-0.04626 b4=0.0925 s11=1.2
s22=1 c12=-1;
xb = b0 + u0 +u01+ b1*Age+b2*LengthofStay+b4*Experience;
p = exp(xb)/(1+exp(xb));
model remission ~ binary(p);
random u0 u01~ normal([0,0],[s11,c12, s22]) subject=DID;
run;
```

Comment Option ABSFCONV helps to get convergence. The clustering is at the doctor's level. There are patients within doctors. We propose that depending on the doctor a patient sees, the remission can be enhanced or delayed. They are not just delivering medication—their input can differ based on certain unknown characteristics. The earlier comments are appropriate for the code when we had the Qpoints option and will not be repeated.

Graphical Representation

The logistic regression model with random effects is represented graphically, where a model with random intercept effects is varying intercepts for each doctor. The model fit above, using Qpoints = 80, is significant random effect, which is seen by the variation in the intercept value of $\log\left(\frac{\hat{P}_{y=1}}{\hat{P}_{y=0}}\right)$, the logit, for each doctor. In Fig. 10.2, the variation in the probability of remission (using the logit) is shown as the age of the patient varies while holding the length of stay and experience at the average values (5.49 and 17.64, respectively). In the random intercept model, the intercept term varies for each doctor, while the slope for age remains constant. We see that the negative slope indicates that the older people are less likely to be in remission.

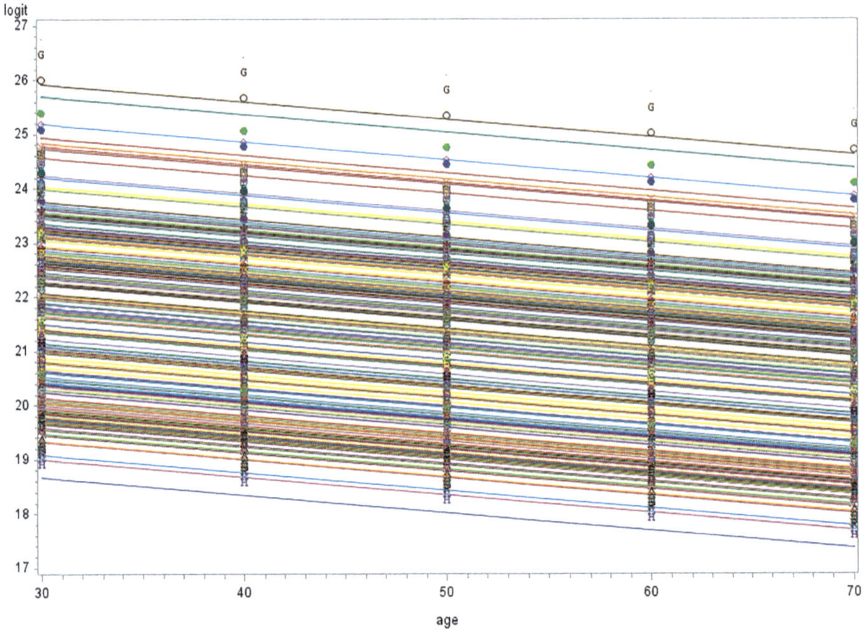

Fig. 10.2 Set of logits plotted versus age

10.5.3 Modeling Random Intercepts for Levels 2 and 3 Using STATA

STATA Program

```
. melogit remission Age LengthofStay Experience  HID:  DID:, nolog
```

STATA Output

```
Mixed-effects logistic regression               Number of obs =  8,525
Grouping information
No. of        Observations per group
Group variable       groups     Minimum     Average     Maximum
HID                   35          134        243.6        377
DID                  407            2         20.9         40
Integration method: mvaghermite              Integration pts.  =     7
Wald chi2(3)    =      184.96
Log-likelihood = -3835.0827                  Prob > chi2   =    0.0000
remission    Coefficient   Std. err.   z   P>z  [95% conf. interval]
Age           -.0325982  .0055345  -5.89 0.000  -.0434455 -.0217508
LengthofStay -.260487   .0330104  -7.89 0.000  -.3251861 -.1957879
```

```
Experience    .1184048   .0256944    4.61 0.000    .0680447   .1687648
_cons        -.4393745   .536119    -0.82 0.412 -1.490149    .6113995
HID
var(_cons)    .2402591   .1442518                  .0740658   .7793671
HID>DID
var(_cons)    3.542232   .3797237                  2.870973   4.370438
LR test vs. logistic model: chi2(2) = 2360.34      Prob > chi2 = 0.0000
```

Note: LR test is conservative and provided only for reference.

Comment The logistic regression model is

$$\log\left(\frac{\hat{P}_{y=1}\,|\text{random effect}}{\hat{P}_{y=0}\,|\text{random effect}}\right) = -0.439 - 0.033\text{Age} - 0.260\text{Los} + 0.118\text{Experience}$$

The variance components s11 and s22 are significant (<0.0001). Thus, the variability among doctors is significant (<0.0001) and the variability among hospitals is significant (<0.0001). It makes good sense to include these random effects. Seeing certain doctors or having stayed at certain hospitals has an impact on patient's remission.

10.5.4 Three-Level Logistic Regression Model with Random Slopes Using SAS

A three-level random intercept and random slope model (10.4) was fitted with both doctors and hospitals as random effects and age of the patient and length of stay as covariates, as well as the experience level of the doctor. We fit these data with two different options: Qpoints = 120 and ABSFCONV = 0.4.

SAS Program

```
proc nlmixed data=HDPDATA  qpoints=120;
parms b0=-3.4462 b1=-0.01128 b2=-0.04626 b4=0.0925  s3u=0.02
s3f=0.003;
randomt= (b2+rb+rbi)*LengthofStay;
xb = b0 + b1*Age+b4*Experience+randomt;
p = exp(xb)/(1+exp(xb)); model remission ~ binary(p);
RANDOM rb rbi~ NORMAL([0,0],[S3U,0,S3F]) SUBJECT=DID;
run;
```

Comment We used PROC NLMIXED with the *Qpoints* option and also with the *ABSFCONV* option. For convergence performance, we fitted the slope as random effects and ignored the intercept. Longford (1993) indicated that for most purposes five-point quadrature suffices. However, for the data, we needed 120 quadrature points. Hartzel et al. (2001) said that the default number of quadrature points in SAS is often inadequate to give proper convergence to ML estimates and their standard errors. They recommended sequential fitting with a successively increasing number of quadrature points until convergence appears to have occurred. We followed their suggestions and used 120. They further stated that for most datasets, however, it is best if the number of clusters is large and not the number of observations within a cluster. We will not repeat comments if they were already made in the chapter for any earlier outputs. We present the results with Qpoints option first.

Parameter estimates

Parameter	Estimate	Standard error	DF	t value	Pr > |t|	Alpha	Lower	Upper	Gradient
b0	0.7054	0.4780	405	1.48	0.1408	0.05	−0.2343	1.6451	−0.00111
b1	−0.03208	0.005518	405	−5.81	<0.0001	0.05	−0.04293	−0.02123	−0.05885
b2	−0.4198	0.03936	405	−10.67	<0.0001	0.05	−0.4972	−0.3425	−0.00243
b4	0.09605	0.02234	405	4.30	<0.0001	0.05	0.05214	0.1400	−0.01537
s3u	0.07659	0.007093	405	10.80	<0.0001	0.05	0.06265	0.09054	−0.00433
s3f	0.05959	0.007093	405	8.40	<0.0001	0.05	0.04565	0.07354	−0.00433

Comment The fitted logistic regression model is

$$\log\left(\frac{\hat{P}_{y=1} \mid \text{random effect}}{\hat{P}_{y=0} \mid \text{random effect}}\right) = -0.705 - 0.032\text{Age} - 0.420\text{Los} + 0.096\text{Experience}$$

where $\hat{\sigma}^2_{hospital}$ =0.076 and $\hat{\sigma}^2_{doctors} = 0.060$. The random slopes have significant variation.

Graphical Representation

The logistic regression model with random effects is represented graphically, where a model with random slopes has varying slopes for each doctor. The model fit above, using Qpoints = 120, has significant random effects that are seen by the variation in the random slope, for each doctor. In Fig. 10.3, the variation in the probability of remission (using the logit) is shown as the length of stay of the patient varies, while holding the age and experience at the average values (5.49 and 17.64, respectively). In the random slope intercept model, the slope varies across doctors, while the slope for age remains constant. We see that the negative slope indicates that the length of stay increased are less likely to be in remission.

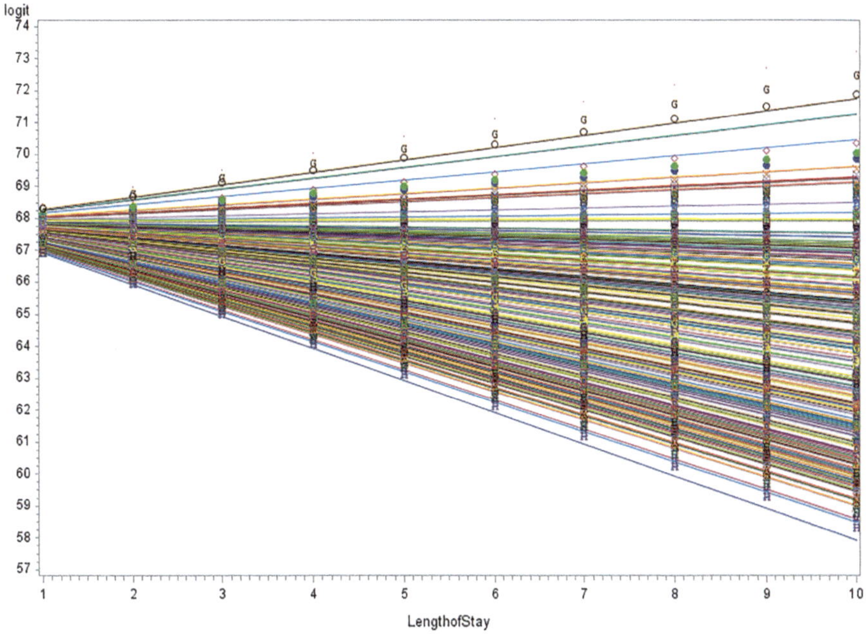

Fig. 10.3 Set of logits plotted versus age

Comment The model fit implies that we had varying rates depending on the length of stay effects. Thus, the differentiated effect that a patient has is also due in part to the doctor, length of stay, and the hospital. The variation is accounted for in the slope for each doctor. In the figure below, it can be seen that the effect of the length of stay affects the probability of remission (using the logit) and varies for each doctor. This can be evaluated by holding age and experience fixed at the average values (50.97 and 17.64, respectively).

10.5.5 Modeling Random Intercepts for Levels 2 and 3 Using R

Code for two random intercepts at the doctor and hospital levels, at levels 2 and 3 using R.

R Program

```
> mremission.true <- glmer(outcome$remission ~ Age + LengthofStay
+ Experience + (1 | DID) + (1 | HID), data = mldat, family =
"binomial")
> print(mremission.true, correlation=FALSE)
> summary(mremission.true)
```

R-Output

Output from print(mremission.true, correlation = FALSE):

```
Generalized linear mixed model fit by maximum likelihood
['glmerMod']
 Family: binomial (logit)
Formula: outcome$remission ~ Age + LengthofStay + Experience + (1
| DID) + (1 | HID)
  Data: mldat
  AIC          BIC                  logLik               deviance
 7770.093     7812.398             -3879.047            7758.093
```

Random effects:

```
Groups       Name              Std.Dev.
DID         (Intercept)       1.8005
HID         (Intercept)       0.3571
Number of obs: 8525, groups: DID, 407; HID, 35
```

Fixed effects:

```
 (Intercept)       Age              LengthofStay           Experience
  -0.78386       -0.02759         -0.22766               0.11471
```

Comment The fixed effects part of the model gives us

$$\log\left(\frac{\hat{P}_{y=1} \mid \text{random effect}}{\hat{P}_{y=0} \mid \text{random effect}}\right) = -0.784 - 0.028\text{Age} - 0.2280\text{Los} + 0.114\text{Experience}$$

The estimate of the parameter associated with doctors' random effect standard error is 1.805 and for hospital is 0.3571. There are 407 doctors and 35 hospitals.

Output from summary(mremission.true):

```
Generalized linear mixed model fit by maximum likelihood
['glmerMod']
Family: binomial ( logit )
Formula: outcome$remission ~ Age + LengthofStay + Experience + (1
| DID) + (1 | HID)
   Data: mldat
 AIC               BIC              logLik              deviance
 7770.093          7812.398         -3879.047           7758.093
```

Comment These are summary statistics about the fit of the model.

Random effects:

```
Groups          Name                    Variance              Std.Dev.
DID            (Intercept)              3.2419                1.8005
HID            (Intercept)              0.1275                0.3571
Number of obs: 8525, groups: DID, 407; HID, 35
```

Comment
The variance and standard deviations of the random effects are given.

Fixed effects:

```
                 Estimate    Std. Error      z value      Pr(>|z|)
(Intercept)     -0.783862     0.520725        -1.505      0.132
Age             -0.027585     0.005007        -5.509      3.61e-08 ***
LengthofStay    -0.227664     0.030617        -7.436      1.04e-13 ***
Experience       0.114707     0.024710         4.642      3.45e-06 ***
---
```

Signif. codes: 0 '***' 0.001 '**' 0.01 '*' 0.05 '.' 0.1 '' 1.

Comment The fixed effects model is

$$\log\left(\frac{\hat{P}_{y=1|\text{random effect}}}{\hat{P}_{y=0|\text{random effect}}}\right) = -0.784 - 0.028\text{Age} - 0.2280\text{Los} + 0.114\text{Experience}$$

The covariates, age, length of stay, and experience are significant in the fixed effects part of the model.

10.5.6 Three-Level Logistic Regression Model with Random Slopes Using R

R Program

```
> mremission.true <- glmer(outcome$remission ~ Age + LengthofStay
+ Experience + (LengthofStay | DID) + (LengthofStay | HID), data
= mldat, family = "binomial")
> print(mremission.true, correlation=FALSE)
> summary(mremission.true)
```

Comment This is the code for two random slopes for Length of Stay predictor at the doctor and hospital levels:

R Output

Output from print(mremission.true, correlation = FALSE):

```
Generalized linear mixed model fit by maximum likelihood
['glmerMod']
 Family: binomial (logit)
Formula: outcome$remission ~ Age + LengthofStay + Experience +
(LengthofStay |      DID) + (LengthofStay | HID)    DID
(Intercept)              0.4425
             LengthofStay              0.2556       1.00
 HID         (Intercept)               0.9496
             LengthofStay              0.1016      -1.00
Number of obs: 8525,     groups: DID, 407;           HID, 35
```

Comment The random effects are given in their standard deviation

Fixed effects:

```
 (Intercept)         Age          LengthofStay           Experience
  -0.15470         -0.02705     -0.33093               0.10668
```

Output from summary(mremission.true):

```
Generalized linear mixed model fit by maximum likelihood
['glmerMod']
 Family: binomial (logit)
Formula: outcome$remission ~ Age + LengthofStay + Experience +
(LengthofStay |      DID) + (LengthofStay | HID)
Data: mldat
AIC                 BIC             logLik              deviance
7744.059            7814.567      -3862.030             7724.059
```

Comment The deviance measures AIC, BIC, loglik, and deviance are meant to address the fit of the model.

Random effects:

Groups	Name	Variance	Std.Dev.	Corr
DID	(Intercept)	0.19580	0.4425	
	LengthofStay	0.06531	0.2556	1.00
HID	(Intercept)	0.90181	0.9496	
	LengthofStay	0.01033	0.1016	-1.00

Number of obs: 8525, groups: DID, 407; HID, 35

Comment An estimate of the variance for the random effects for the intercept and the slopes are given.

Fixed effects:

	Estimate	Std. Error	z value	Pr(>|z|)	
(Intercept)	-0.154702	0.514271	-0.301	0.764	
Age	-0.027054	0.005024	-5.385	7.23e-08	***
LengthofStay	-0.330928	0.038185	-8.666	< 2e-16	***
Experience	0.106684	0.022956	4.647	3.36e-06	***

Signif. codes: 0 '***' 0.001 '**' 0.01 '*' 0.05 '.' 0.1 '' 1.

Comment From the fixed effects part of the model, age, length of stay, and experience of the model are significant factors.

Correlation of fixed effects:

	(Intr)	Age	LngthS
Age	-0.397		
LengthofSty	-0.297	-0.227	
Experience	-0.800	-0.006	0.023

10.5.7 Three-Level Logistic Regression Model with Random Slopes at Doctor Level Using STATA

STATA Program

```
melogit remission Age LengthofStay Experience || HID: || DID:
LengthofStay,
```

STATA Output

```
Mixed-effects logistic regression Number of obs = 8,525
        Grouping information
----------------------------------------------------------------
          |      No. of       Observations per group
  Group variable |      groups    Minimum     Average     Maximum
-------------------+--------------------------------------------
       HID |              35         134       243.6         377
       DID |             407           2        20.9          40
----------------------------------------------------------------
Integration method: mvaghermite            Integration pts.   =    7
                    Wald chi2(3)        =       194.57
Log likelihood = -3818.2077                 Prob > chi2    =  0.0000
------------------------------------------------------------------
remission | Coefficient  Std. err.    z      P>|z|     [95% conf. interval]
-------------+----------------------------------------------------
Age |    -.0324081  .0055575  -5.83  0.000  -.0433006  -.0215157
LengthofStay | -.3828525  .043052    -8.89  0.000    -.4672328
-.2984722
Experience | .1077718  .0240137   4.49  0.000  .0607058  .1548377
_cons |        .3513355  .535272    0.66  0.51  -.6977784 1.400449
-------------+----------------------------------------------------
HID                   |
    var(_cons)|   .4247219   .1789008             .1860213   .9697208
-------------+----------------------------------------------------
HID>DID               |
var(Lengtho~y)|   .1006019   .0210589             .0667459   .1516308
    var(_cons)|   .6856626   .5071397             .1608913   2.922055
------------------------------------------------------------------
LR test vs. logistic model: chi2(3) = 2394.09        Prob > chi2 = 0.0000
```

Note: LR test is conservative and provided only for reference.

10.5.8 Interpretation

The interpretations of the coefficients in the generalized linear mixed model are somewhat similar to the logic we used in Chap. 3 and the standard logistic regression model. Whenever we use the logit link, we are on a linear scale, but on the original scale (the inverse link function), there is no longer linearity scale. On the original scale, we can talk about the probability of an outcome given some specific values of the predictors. This means that the random intercepts are additive on link but have a multiplicative effect on probabilities.

Binary Outcomes

Consider the hierarchical logistic model, predicting remission (yes = 1, no = 0) from length of stay and experience. We allow the slopes to vary randomly for each doctor and slopes to vary for each hospital. Essentially, the estimates can be interpreted as usual for binary outcome data. For example, for age, a one unit increase in age is associated with a 0.032 unit decrease in the expected log odds of remission. In a random effects model, the odds ratios are not the same as in the fixed effects model. In the fixed effects model, the odds ratios are the expected odds ratio while holding all or other predictors fixed. As for the mixed effects logistic models, there is the addition of holding the random effect fixed. At this point, one might be wondering how to keep the random effect fixed. The odds ratio in the mixed model is a conditional odds ratio. It is either the same doctor or doctors with the same random effects. However, when there is large variability between doctors, the relative impact of the fixed effects may be decimated. In such situations, researchers have suggested that one should examine the effects at various levels of the random effects or to get the average fixed effects and average out the random effects.

10.6 Conclusions

It is not a new phenomenon that a statistical model should reflect the design and the method whereby the data were collected. There seem to be multiple sources of variation, and thus, the hierarchical structures inherent in the data are addressed. In particular, in the data analyzed there is the variation due to the clustering of observations from the same doctor and doctors from the same hospital. As such, we address the variation between doctors through a random effect, as well as the variation between hospitals with another random effect. We analyze these data through taking different levels of nesting into account when we addressed factors impacting the outcome.

There was the variation between doctors taken as a random effect as well as the variation between hospitals also taken as random effect. Using the standard binomial logistic regression model would ignore several sources of variation. However, the hierarchical logistic regression model incorporates these different sources of variation. We fit a nested three-level logistic regression model with random intercept and with random intercepts and random slopes. One may encounter challenges with convergence. With these added parameters and inherent covariance matrices, there may be challenges with convergence. The SAS procedures outlined in this chapter provide a practical guide for evaluating nested three-level models and higher with binary outcomes. One of the challenges to fitting these models in the SAS NLMIXED procedure is the use of quadrature points. This becomes increasingly difficult when there are higher levels of nesting. The best starting values are those obtained from the attempted fit of any logistic regression model. Lesaffre and Spiessens said they are aware of the dependence of the outcome of a logistic random effects model on the number of quadrature points. They said that in MIXOR, Q = 10 (i.e., 10 quadrature points) is often sufficient, and when differences are found by increasing Q, they are minimal. They believe that the Gauss-Hermite method robustly calculates the subject-specific estimates of the parameters and did not need a routine check, as opposed to the methods on which the SAS macro GLIMMIX is based. They are pleased to see that adaptive Gaussian quadrature can be used in NLMIXED. However, we share the experience that, even with adaptive Gaussian quadrature, increased points, and relatively simple models, convergence to a global maximum can be difficult to obtain. This continues to emphasize the computational difficulties with random effects models for binary outcome data at higher levels of nesting.

Both the random intercepts model and the random intercepts and random slopes model can be fitted with PROC NLMIXED. The NLMIXED procedure maximizes the likelihood directly by numerical integration methods and adaptive Gaussian quadrature (Kuss, 2002). We obtained exact maximum likelihood estimates of the parameters when the number of quadrature points was large enough.

10.7 Related Examples

In his dissertation, Subedi (2004) used data taken from the National Assessment of Educational Progress (NAEP). The subjects were students in the fourth grade. The sample he used was formed by 7175 students, 1076 teachers, and 295 schools. The primary purpose of this study was to demonstrate that hierarchical generalized linear models can be applied to research in education, by measuring the reading proficiency of students in fourth grade. The response variable was binary, with reading proficiency or non-proficiency as the outcome. The data were leveled in the following way: student, teacher, and school represented level 1, level 2, and level 3, respectively. In this study, not only student-level variables were taken into account, but also teacher-level and school-level predictors were taken into account. This is an example of students nested within teachers nested within schools. Since the outcome is binary, a hierarchical logistic regression model could be used for this analysis. The citation for this work is Subedi, B.R. (2004). *A demonstration of the three-level hierarchical generalized linear model applied to educational research. Electronic* The link to this dissertation is: Diginole.lib.fsu.edu/cgi/viewcontent.cgi?article = 4896&context = etd.

References

Austin, P. C. (2010). Estimating multilevel logistic regression models when the number of clusters is low: A comparison of different statistical software procedures. *The International Journal of Biostatistics, 6*(1), 1–20.

Hartzel, J., Agresti, A., & Caffo, B. (2001). Multinomial logit random effects models. *Statistical Modelling, 1*(2), 81–102.
Hedeker, D., Mermelstein, R. J., & Demirtas, H. (2008). An application of a mixed effects location scale model for analysis of ecological momentary assessment (EMA) data. *Biometrics, 64*(2), 627–634.
Hedeker, D., Mermelstein, R. J., & Demirtas, H. (2012). Modeling between- and within subject variance in ecological momentary assessment (EMA) data using mixed-effects location scale models. *Statistics in Medicine, 31*(27), 3328–3336.
Kuss, O. (2002). How to use SAS® for logistic regression with correlated data. In *SUGI 27 Proceedings*, 261-27.
Longford, N. T. (1993). *Random coefficient models*. Clarendon.
Maas, C. J. M., & Hox, J. J. (2004). The influence of violations of assumptions on multilevel parameter estimates and their standard errors. *Computational Statistics & Data Analysis, 46*(3), 427–440.
McMahon, J. M., Pouget, E. R., & Tortu, S. (2006). A guide for multilevel modeling of dyadic data with binary outcomes using SAS PROC NLMIXED. *Computational Statistics & Data Analysis, 50*(12), 3663–3680.
Newsom, J. T. (2002). A multilevel structural equation model for dyadic data. *Structural Equation Modeling: A Multidisciplinary Journal, 9*(3), 431–447.
Rasbash, J., Steele, F., Browne, W. J., & Goldstein, H. (2012). *User's guide to WLwiN, version 2.26*. Centre for Multilevel Modelling, University of Bristol. Retrieved from http://www.bristol.ac.uk/cmm/software/mlwin/download/2-26/manual-web.pdf
Raudenbush, S. W. (1992). *Hierarchical linear models*. Sage.
Rodriquez, G., & Goldman, N. (1995). An assessment of estimation procedures for multilevel models with binary responses. *Journal of the Royal Statistical Society, Series A (Statistics in Society), 158*(1), 73–89.
Schabenberger, O. (2005). Introducing the GLIMMIX procedure for generalized linear mixed models. In *SUGI 30 proceedings*, 196-30.
Shahian, D. M., Normand, S. L., Torchiana, D. F., Lewis, S. M., Pastore, J. O., Kuntz, R. E., et al. (2001). Cardiac surgery report cards: Comprehensive review and statistical critique. *The Annals of Thoracic Surgery, 72*(6), 2155–2168.
Subedi, B. (2004). Emerging Trends of Research on Transfer of Learning. *International Education Journal, 5*.
Wedderburn, R. W. M. (1974). Quasi-likelihood functions, generalized linear models and the Gauss-Newton method. *Biometrika, 61*(3), 439–447.

Chapter 11
Fixed Effects Logistic Regression Model

11.1 Motivating Example

We are often reminded in our introductory statistics courses that we should talk about relationships rather than cause and effects when we analyze observational data (Sobel, 2000). At times, the beginner to data analysis wonders about this statement, and even though they are faced with examples, they are often puzzled to accept it. Beginners are equally puzzled when posed with the thought of unmeasured covariates. In a control experiment, can we control for covariates that have not been measured? Or can we account for covariates that cannot be measured?

In sociology and in particular the study of juvenile delinquency, it is common to hear one wants to know whether watching violent television programs increases delinquency among teenagers. It is intuitive to think that one compares an individual's delinquency rate when he/she is watching violent television programs with his/her delinquency rate when he/she is not. The difference in delinquency rates between the two cases is an estimate of the television effect for that individual. Or, one might see how a child's performance in school differs depending on how much time he/she spends playing video games. So, one compares how the child does when spending significant time playing video games versus when he/she does not play video games. If these factors are possible and measurable, one can use the fixed effects and hence test the mean difference. In such cases for binary responses, we consider fixed effects logistic regression models. In general, fixed effects logistic regression models are useful to analyze longitudinal data with repeated measures on both the response and the covariates. In fixed effects models, we focus on what is measured. While in random effects models, the focus is on what cannot be measured.

Substantively, fixed effects models are designed to study the causes of changes within a person [or entity]. A time-invariant characteristic cannot cause such a change, because it is constant for each person (Kohler & Kreuter, 2012).

J. R. Wilson et al., *Modeling Binary Correlated Responses*, ICSA Book Series in Statistics, https://doi.org/10.1007/978-3-031-62427-8_11

11.2 Definition and Notation

A *fixed effects* logistic regression model (with repeated measures on the covariates) treats unobserved differences between individuals as a set of fixed parameters that can either be directly estimated or canceled out. *Fixed effects* estimates are obtained within-individual differences, and as such, any information about differences between individuals is now excluded and unavailable for estimation (Allison, 2005).

In Chap. 9, we introduced a *random effects* model. For such models, the unobserved differences are treated as random variables with a specified probability distribution, usually the normal distribution. In such models, the unobserved random variables are assumed to be uncorrelated with all the observed variables. However, the random effects model estimates information from both within and between individuals (Wooldridge, 2002).

Conditional maximum likelihood estimation is an alternative to full-information maximum likelihood estimation. Not all the parameters are unknown. Thus, the maximization problem is simplified, as there are fewer parameters to be estimated. As some of these parameters are given certain values, the maximization is on the conditional log-likelihood function.

Conditional maximum likelihood estimates are consistent but are said to be less efficient. They are found to be most useful when the full log-likelihood function is difficult or impossible to derive or maximize.

Subject-specific models or random-effects models assume that the relationship between the response and the covariate differs between subjects. They tell about the individual.

Population-averaged or marginal models assume that the relationship between the response and the covariate is the same for all subjects. They tell about the mean of the population.

11.3 Exploratory Analysis

11.3.1 Philippine's Data

We choose to revisit the Philippines' data first analyzed by Lai and Small (2007). These data were collected by the International Food Policy Research Institute in the Bukidnon Province in the Philippines and focused on quantifying the association between body mass index (BMI) and morbidity 4 months into the future. Data were collected at four-time points, separated by 4-month intervals (Bhargava, 1994). There are 370 children with three observations each. The covariates are as follows: BMI, age, gender, and time as categorical variables and represented by two indicator variables. The data are modeled, and the sickness intensity is measured by adding the duration of sicknesses and taking a logistic transformation of the proportion of time for which a child is sick with a continuity correction for extreme values.

As it is well-known among researchers, through the use of experimental research designs, those unmeasured differences between subjects can often be accounted for through the use of randomly assigned treatment and control groups (Allison, 2005). However, in the analysis of repeated measures data, when a subject is measured at two or more points in time, we consider the subject to be under their own control. Therefore, when analyzing longitudinal data, we control for characteristics that do not change across time whether they are measured or not. Such characteristics include demographic variables, such as race, gender, ethnicity, intelligence, and genetic makeup. However, Allison tells us there are basically two conditions under which one may use a fixed effects logistic regression model:

1. The response is repeatedly observed for each individual. So, an individual is a cluster.
2. The covariate is time-dependent. So, the covariate value changes across time for some significant proportion of the subjects/units. In general, such covariates fall mostly into one of three categories:
   (a) Covariates are unobservable.
   (b) Covariates are observable but do not change over time.
   (c) Covariates are observable but do change over time.

When using a fixed effects logistic regression model, the unobserved variables are basically treated as fixed parameters. In Chaps. 9 and 10, we treat the unobserved effects as random. In the fixed effects logistic regression model, we make use of the variables that change over time. Thus, fixed effects models do not produce any estimates of variable effects that are time-independent. Some researchers have shown that the estimates may have substantially larger standard errors than random effect estimates and, as such, lead to higher p-values and hence wider confidence intervals (Allison, 2005).

11.4 Statistical Models

A fixed effects logistic regression model is used to analyze data when there are repeated measures of the response and the covariates are time-dependent. In fact:

(i) It treats each measurement on each subject as a separate observation.
(ii) It operates as a conditional model also referred to as a subject-specific model as opposed to being a population-averaged model.
(iii) It has the ability to control for all fixed characteristics (time-independent) of the individuals.
(iv) It applies to those measured or not (Allison, 2005).
(v) It uses only within-individual variation to estimate the regression coefficients.
(vi) It implies that the set of subject coefficients would be eliminated through conditional methods (Allison, 2005).

Allison pointed out that a strength of a fixed effects model is the fact that the effects of stable characteristics, such as race and gender, are controlled for, whether they are measured or not. However, the challenge is that the effects of these omitted variables are not able to be estimated. While the omitted variables are not explicitly measured as they are controlled for, their effects are not estimated.

Fixed effects model estimates are based on *only within-individual differences*, as they ignore the between individuals. The fixed effects model estimates are less accurate with larger standard errors than if subjects only had between differences as opposed to within. The effects of the omitted variable are better addressed by models other than fixed effects. Moreover, there is a trade-off between bias and efficiency. Other models, such as the random effects models (Chaps. 9 and 10), suffer from omitted variable bias.

Fixed effects logistic regression models help to control for omitted variable bias by having individuals serve as their own control, while random effects models help with efficiency. In short, we see from Table 11.1, a comparison of models regarding bias and efficiency. It shows that for fixed effect there is less bias and less efficiency, but random effects models are more biased but more efficiency. However, fixed effects will not control for unobserved (omitted variable) time-dependent covariates. As such, the type of variable omitted helps in its determination.

The fundamental principle of the fixed effects model is about differences between time-periods. Suppose we averaged those differences across all persons in the population, we would obtain an estimate of the average "treatment effect." In so doing, such a procedure will, through averaging over time, be controlling for time-independent factors. While it does not control for time-dependent variables, these can be handled by including them in a regression model. There are two basic data requirements for using fixed effects methods.

11.4.1 Fixed Effects Regression Models with Two Observations Per Unit

We fit a fixed effects logistic regression model for the case when there are two observations per unit. Consider observation obtained on the same unit on two successive time-periods. If we were to fit the standard logistic regression at each time, then we can answer questions about the response for each of two occasions. Then, we write for unit/subject *i*, at time (1) and at time (2), respectively, as

$$\log\left(\frac{p_{i(1)}}{1-p_{i(1)}}\right)=\beta_0+\beta_1 X_{i1}+\beta_2 X_{i2}+\gamma_1 W_{i1(1)}+\gamma_2 W_{i2(1)}+\tau_{i(1)}$$

Table 11.1 Bias and efficiency and fixed versus random effects model

	Bias	Efficiency
Fixed effects model	− ↓	− ↓
Random effects model	+ ↑	+ ↑

$$\log\left(\frac{p_{i(2)}}{1-p_{i(2)}}\right) = \beta_0 + \beta_1 X_{i1} + \beta_2 X_{i2} + \gamma_1 W_{i1(2)} + \gamma_2 W_{i2(2)} + \tau_{i(2)}$$

where β_0 denotes an intercept that varies with time for all units (type of average), β_1 is a regression coefficient related to the known X_1, and β_2 is a regression coefficient related to the known X_2, where X_1 and X_2 are variables, whose values remain the same over time. The covariates W_1 and W_2 are variables, whose values change over time, and γ_1 and γ_2 are regression coefficients associated with W_1 and W_2. The τ_i represents unobserved covariates for each person that are not represented by W_1 and W_2. Subtracting the equations for time (1) from time (2) gives

$$\log\left\{\left(\frac{p_{i(2)}}{1-p_{i(2)}}\right)\Big/\left(\frac{p_{i(1)}}{1-p_{i(1)}}\right)\right\} = \left\{\gamma_1 W_{i1(2)} - \gamma_1 W_{i2(1)}\right\} + \left\{\gamma_2 W_{i1(2)} - \gamma_2 W_{i2(1)}\right\}$$

since X_i remains the same. The left side is equivalent to $\log\left\{\left(\frac{\left(1-p_{i(1)}\right)p_{i(2)}}{\left(1-p_{i(2)}\right)p_{i(1)}}\right)\right\}$, which is the log of the ratio of the joint probability of nonevent on time 1 multiplied by the probability of an event on time 2, to joint probability of event on time 1 multiplied by the probability of nonevent on time 2. The left side represents those cases where the outcomes are different. We have in effect decreased the sample to concentrate only on subjects whose responses have changed from time 1 to time 2. The right side is the difference; however, variables with the same values are canceled out. In fact, the analysis concentrates on those units with different outcomes on the responses. The right-hand side now becomes the change in time-dependent covariates. We can look upon this as a logistic regression model on a smaller dataset. In fact, if we ignore covariate, this is the same as McNemar's test.

In order to analyze the data with two observations per subject, we will fit the model on the data where there are different responses from time 1 to time 2 and instead consider:

$$\text{logit}\left\{p_{i(2)}\right\} = \left\{\beta_{0(2)} - \beta_{0(1)}\right\} + \gamma_1\left\{W_{i1(2)} - W_{i1(1)}\right\} + \gamma_2\left\{W_{i2(2)} - W_{i2(1)}\right\} + \beta_1 X_{i1} + \beta_2 X_{i2} \tag{11.1}$$

The function e^{γ_1} or e^{γ_2} based on the change in covariates is interpreted as usual, the odds ratio with unit change. However, the interpretation of the odds ratio e^{β_1} or e^{β_2} based on the covariates that do not change is not as clear. In fact, e^{β_1} is the odds of an event in time for a unit change in X_1. Similarly, e^{β_2} is the odds of an event in time for a unit change in X_2. Thus, we can consider X_1 and X_2 as interaction variable interactions between the actual predictor and time. They can be best explained in Table 11.2. Consider $W_1 = 3$ at $t = t$ and $t = t + 1$, $W_2 = 11$ at $t = t$ and $t = t + 1$ also let $X_1 = 4$, $X_2 = 5$ and 6.

Table 11.2 Example of interpretation of variables

	W_1	W_2	X_1	X_2
i = i t = t	3	11	4	5
i = i t = t + 1	3	11	4	5
i = r t = t	3	11	4	6
i = r t = t + 1	3	11	4	6

11.4.2 Modeling More Than Two Observations Per Unit: Conditional Logistic Regression Model

In this section, we will refer a great deal to the conditional logistic regression model. Think of the data broken up into small groups or strata based on some factor or factors. We will not necessarily use all the observations but just the cases where the outcome has changed for at least one of the occasions in which they were observed. So, the final analysis is done on a subset of the original data. Thus, the questions being answered may be related but not exactly as if the full dataset was used.

When there are more than two observations per unit, we can use conditional logistic regression (CLR) (Agresti, 2007). Conditional logistic regression is, in fact, a standard logistic regression applied to a particular segment of the data. In particular, this method of analysis is used when the data occur in clusters where at least one of the observations is the event. Then, we wish to condition the number of events within a group. Hence, we are fitting a logistic regression model to explain how observation 1 had an event in group 1 conditioned on one of the observations in the group having an event. In fact, we fit a model that explains how observation 1 had an event in group 1, observation 3 had an event in group 2, and so on (Harris et al., 1999). If we assumed the unconditional probability of a positive outcome could be explained by the standard logistic model, then the standard logistic regression model is not an appropriate model for our data because it does not account for the conditioning. The two models are answering different questions. One model uses a subset of the data, while the other uses the full dataset. This conditional model explains how an event occurred or the odds of the event occurring. Therefore, we have a model fit such that

$$Prob\{Event\ and\ Nonevent|Event\} = \frac{\exp\left(\gamma_1 W_{i1(1)} + \gamma_2 W_{i2(1)}\right)}{\exp\left(\gamma_1 W_{i1(1)} + \gamma_2 W_{i2(1)}\right) + \exp\left(\gamma_1 W_{i1(2)} + \gamma_2 W_{i2(2)}\right)}$$

For a thorough discussion of the conditional logistic derivation and its implications, see Harris et al., (1999). Groups that contain all-positive or all-negative outcomes provide no information because the conditional probability of observing such groups is 1 regardless of the values of the regression parameters. Thus, when the process of analysis encounters such groups, it reports that so many groups were dropped "due to all positive or all negative outcomes."

11.5 Analysis of Data

11.5.1 Fixed Effects Logistic Regression Model with Two Observations Per Unit

We first fit the fixed effects logistic regression model with two observations per child through differencing. Later, we fit a model for four time-points per person using conditional maximum likelihood. We fit a fixed effects logistic regression model with two observations per unit to the Philippines' data for time-periods 2 and 3 (Table 11.3). We use SAS, SPSS, R, and STATA.

The identification of the child in the dataset is represented as *Childid.* There are other variables as in *BMI, age*, and *gender*. *Time* denotes the period. *T1, T2,* and *T3* are the binary variables derived from *time. Sick* is the binary response that we model.

Table 11.3 Partial dataset from the Philippines

Childid	BMI	Age	Gender	Time	t1	t2	t3	Sick	Status
206	14.95	59.27	0	1	1	0	0	0	0
206	15.02	63.40	0	2	0	1	0	0	0
206	14.79	66.83	0	3	0	0	1	0	0
407	18.08	25.07	0	3	0	0	1	0	1
407	17.02	17.50	0	1	1	0	0	1	1
407	16.01	21.67	0	2	0	1	0	1	1
705	15.09	70.17	1	3	0	0	1	0	1
705	15.83	62.60	1	1	1	0	0	0	1
705	15.39	66.77	1	2	0	1	0	1	1
1105	16.07	29.03	1	2	0	1	0	1	0
1105	17.73	25.00	1	1	1	0	0	1	0
1105	15.94	32.53	1	3	0	0	1	1	0
.	.	.	.	.	.	.	.	.	.
.	.	.	.	.	.	.	.	.	.

11.5.2 *Fixed Effects Logistic Regression Model with Two Observations Per Unit Using SAS*

SAS Program

```
DATA mydata; SET philippb; RUN;
TITLE 'Reshape long data into wide data';
PROC SORT DATA=mydata OUT=mydatasort;
  BY childid; RUN;
DATA mydatawide; SET mydatasort;
  BY childid;
  KEEP childid sick1-sick3 BMI1-BMI3 age1-age3 gender;
  RETAIN sick1-sick3 BMI1-BMI3 age1-age3;
  ARRAY asick(1:3) sick1-sick3;
  ARRAY aBMI(1:3)  BMI1-BMI3;
  ARRAY aage(1:3)  age1-age3;
  IF first.childid THEN
  DO;
    DO i = 1 to 3 ;
          asick( i ) = .;
      aBMI( i ) = . ;
      aage( i ) = . ;
    END;
  END;
  asick( time ) = sick;
  aBMI( time ) = BMI ;
  aage( time ) = age ;
  IF last.childid THEN OUTPUT; RUN;
TITLE2 'Using t=2 and t=3 observations for illustration'; * N=134;
DATA mydatadif3; SET mydatawide;
IF sick2 = sick3 THEN DELETE;
BMI = BMI3-BMI2; age = age3-age2; RUN;

PROC FREQ DATA=mydatadif3; TABLES sick3*gender / LIST; RUN;
PROC LOGISTIC DATA=mydatadif3 DESCEND; MODEL sick3 = BMI age
gender; RUN;
```

childid	BMI	age	gender	time	t1	t2	t3	sick	status
206	14.95059	59.26667	0	1	1	0	0	0	0
206	15.01923	63.4	0	2	0	1	0	0	0
206	14.79053	66.83334	0	3	0	0	1	0	0
407	18.08021	25.06667	0	3	0	0	1	0	1
407	17.02125	17.5	0	1	1	0	0	1	1

childid	BMI	age	gender	time	t1	t2	t3	sick	status
407	16.0064	21.66667	0	2	0	1	0	1	1
705	15.08541	70.16666	1	3	0	0	1	0	1
705	15.83377	62.6	1	1	1	0	0	0	1
705	15.39259	66.76667	1	2	0	1	0	1	1
1105	16.07259	29.03333	1	2	0	1	0	1	0
1105	17.7297	25	1	1	1	0	0	1	0
1105	15.9375	32.53333	1	3	0	0	1	1	0
1207	14.51247	75.13333	0	3	0	0	1	0	1
1207	14.66714	71.56667	0	2	0	1	0	0	1
1207	14.76285	67.56667	0	1	1	0	0	1	1
1304	17.61792	25.13333	1	3	0	0	1	0	0
1304	18.9726	17.56667	1	1	1	0	0	0	0
1304	15.14514	21.56667	1	2	0	1	0	0	0
.	.	.	.	.	.	.	.	.	.
.	.	.	.	.	.	.	.	.	.
.	.	.	.	.	.	.	.	.	.
	.	.	.	.	.	.	.	.	.

Comment We fit the conditional model

$$\operatorname{logit}\left(Probability_{event\ at\ time\ 3}\right) = \beta_0 + \beta_1\mathrm{BMI}_1 + \beta_2\mathrm{Age}_2 + \gamma_1\mathrm{Gender}_3$$

Covariates age and BMI represent the difference between year 2 and year 3. Gender is a time-independent covariate.

SAS Output

Using time = 2 and time = 3 observations for illustration

The FREQ procedure

Sick3	Gender	Frequency	Percent	Cumulative frequency	Cumulative percent
0	0	23	17.16	23	17.16
0	1	28	20.90	51	38.06
1	0	43	32.09	94	70.15
1	1	40	29.85	134	100.00

Comment During time-period 3, we had 134 useable observations, where both outcomes are different during periods 2 and 3.

The LOGISTIC procedure	
Model information	
DataSet	WORK.MYDATADIF3
Response variable	Sick3
Number of response levels	2
Model	Binary logit
Optimization technique	Fisher's scoring
Number of observations read	134
Number of observations used	134

Response profile		
Ordered value	Sick3	Total frequency
1	1	83
2	0	51

Comment Fisher's scoring is an iterative reweighted least squares method for obtaining parameter estimates and based on the expected information matrix. This subset of data consists of 134 observations. There were 83 observations with a "1" response in time = 3. We have excluded 370–134 = 236 subjects as they had values "0 and 0" and "1 and 1" as opposed to "1 and 0" or "0 and 1."

Probability modeled is sick3 = 1		
Model convergence status		
Convergence criterion (GCONV = 1E-8) satisfied		
Model fit statistics		
Criterion	Intercept only	Intercept and covariates
AIC	180.047	185.411
SC	182.945	197.002
−2 Log L	178.047	177.411

Comment These fit statistics gives the values with the intercept only and with the covariates included. The difference gives the significance of the covariates.

Testing global null hypothesis: Beta = 0			
Test	Chi-Square	DF	Pr > ChiSq
Likelihood ratio	0.6363	3	0.8881
Score	0.6351	3	0.8883
Wald	0.6336	3	0.8887

Comment These values (likelihood ratio, score, and Wald) talk about the significance of the covariates.

Analysis of maximum likelihood estimates					
Parameter	DF	Estimate	Standard error	Wald Chi-Square	Pr > ChiSq
Intercept	1	−0.5033	4.4260	0.0129	0.9095
BMI	1	0.0105	0.1377	0.0058	0.9391
Age	1	0.3302	1.2935	0.0652	0.7985
Gender	1	−0.2789	0.3627	0.5913	0.4419

Comment Neither BMI (p = 0.9391), age (p = 0.7985), or gender (p = 0.4419) was significant. The fitted model equation is

$$\text{logit}\left(Probability_{event\,at\,time3}\right) = -0.503 + 0.011\text{BMI} + 0.330\text{Age} - 0.279\text{Gender}$$

Odds ratio estimates			
Effect	Point estimate	95% Wald confidence limits	
BMI	1.011	0.772	1.324
Age	1.391	0.110	17.557
Gender	0.757	0.372	1.540

Comment The odds ratio has confidence intervals that all cover the value of 1. So, the variables (BMI, age, and gender) are not significant in the model.

11.5.3 Fixed Effects Logistic Regression Model with Two Observations Per Unit Using SPSS

SPSS

Conditional logistic regression models are designed for situations in which one or more "cases," which show the response of interest, are matched with one or more "controls," which do not show the response. This can be done in the NOMREG procedure, which is accessed in the menus via Analyze>Regression>Multinomial Logistic, (SPSS Advanced Statistical Procedures Companion, by Marija Norusis). http://www-01.ibm.com/support/docview.wss?uid=swg21477360

SPSS Program

```
NOMREG sick3 (BASE=LAST ORDER=ASCENDING) WITH BMI Age gender
  /CRITERIA CIN(95) DELTA(0) MXITER(100) MXSTEP(5) CHKSEP(20)
LCONVERGE(0) PCONVERGE(0.000001) SINGULAR(0.00000001)
  /MODEL
  /STEPWISE=PIN(.05) POUT(0.1) MINEFFECT(0) RULE(SINGLE)
ENTRYMETHOD(LR) REMOVALMETHOD(LR)
  /INTERCEPT=INCLUDE
  /PRINT=PARAMETER SUMMARY LRT CPS STEP MFI.
```

SPSS Output

Case processing summary

	N	Marginal percentage	
Sick3	0	51	38.1%
	1	83	61.9%
Valid		134	100.0%
Missing		0	
Total		134	
Subpopulation		134[a]	

[a]The dependent variable has only one value observed in 134 (100.0%) subpopulations

Model fitting information

Model	Model fitting criteria	Likelihood ratio tests		
	−2 Log likelihood	Chi-Square	DF	Sig.
Intercept only	178.047			
Final	177.411	0.636	3	0.888
Pseudo R-square				
Cox and Snell	0.005			
Nagelkerke	0.006			
McFadden	0.004			

Comment This is the pseudo R^2. It plays a similar role as R^2 in linear models. The values here are very small, suggesting that the model is not a good fit.

Likelihood ratio tests

Effect	Model fitting criteria	Likelihood ratio tests		
	−2 Log-likelihood of reduced model	Chi-square	DF	Sig.
Intercept	177.424	0.013	1	0.909
BMI	177.417	0.006	1	0.939
Age	177.476	0.065	1	0.798
Gender	178.004	0.593	1	0.441

Comment The chi-square statistic is the difference in −2 log-likelihoods between the final model and a reduced model. The reduced model is formed by omitting an effect from the final model. The null hypothesis is that all parameters of that effect are 0.

Parameter estimates

Sick3[a]		B	Std. error	Wald	DF	Sig.	Exp(B)	95% confidence interval for Exp(B)	
								Lower bound	Upper bound
0	Intercept	0.503	4.426	0.013	1	0.909			
	BMI	−0.011	0.138	0.006	1	0.939	0.990	0.755	1.296
	Age	−0.330	1.294	0.065	1	0.799	0.719	0.057	9.071
	Gender	0.279	0.363	0.591	1	0.442	1.322	0.649	2.691

[a]The reference category is 1

Comment Neither BMI (p = 0.939), age (p = 0.799), or gender (p = 0.442) was significant. The model equation is

$$\text{logit}\left(Probability_{event\ at\ time3}\right) = -0.503 + 0.011\text{BMI} + 0.330\text{Age} - 0.279\text{Gender}$$

11.5.4 Fixed Effects Logistic Regression Model with Two Observations Per Unit Using R

R Program

```
> glm.out=glm(formula = sick3 ~ BMI + age + gender, family =
binomial(link=logit), data = data1)
> summary(glm.out)
Call:
glm(formula = sick3 ~ BMI + age + gender, family = binomial(link
= logit),
    data = data1)
```

R Output

```
Deviance Residuals:
Min       1Q        Median    3Q        Max
-1.4839   -1.3352   0.9186    1.0209    1.0760
```

Comment The deviance residuals are as small as −1.4839 and the maximum as large as 1.0760 and median 0.9186. The first quartile is −1.3352 and the third quartile is 1.0209.

```
Coefficients:
              Estimate     Std. Error    z value     Pr(>|z|)
(Intercept)   -0.50334     4.42600       -0.114      0.909
BMI            0.01052     0.13770        0.076      0.939
age            0.33018     1.29354        0.255      0.799
gender        -0.27891     0.36271       -0.769      0.442
```

Comment The fitted model is

$$\text{logit}\left(Probability_{event\,at\,time3}\right) = -0.503 + 0.011\text{BMI}_1 + 0.330\text{Age}_2 - 0.279\ \text{Gender}$$

(Dispersion parameter for binomial family taken to be 1)
Null deviance: 178.05 on 133 degrees of freedom.
Residual deviance: 177.41 on 130 degrees of freedom.
AIC: 185.41.
Number of Fisher scoring iterations: 4.

Comment Measure on the fit of the covariates in the model is measured by 178.05 with no covariates and 177.41 is the measure with three (BMI, age, and gender) covariates.

11.5.5 Fixed Effects Logistic Regression Model with Two Observations Per Unit Using STATA

STATA Program

```
clogit sick bmi age t2, group(childid)
```

STATA Output

```
note: multiple positive outcomes within groups encountered.
note: 236 groups (472 obs) omitted because of all positive or
all negative outcomes.
Iteration 0:  Log-likelihood = -92.591269
Iteration 1:  Log-likelihood = -89.039952
Iteration 2:  Log-likelihood = -89.002218
Iteration 3:  Log-likelihood = -89.002217
Conditional (fixed effects) logistic regression     Number of obs =268
                      LR chi2(3)     = 7.76
                      Prob > chi2    = 0.0513
Log-likelihood = -89.002217                       Pseudo R2   = 0.0418
sick | Coefficient  Std. err.    z     P>|z|     [95% conf. interval]
bmi  |  .0212375    .1371196   0.15   0.877     -.247512     .2899869
age  |  .2077927    1.277272   0.16   0.871     -2.295614  2.711199
t2   |  .2269889    4.390073   0.05   0.959     -8.377397    8.831375
```

Comment Neither BMI (p = 0.877) or age (p = 0.871) was significant.

11.6 Fixed Effects Logistic Regression Model with More Than Two Observations

We fit a fixed effects logistic regression model. In this analysis, we analyze a complete set of data with three time-periods of repeated measures using the conditional logistic regression model.

11.6.1 Fixed Effects Logistic Regression Model with More Than Two Observations Using SAS

SAS Program

```
DATA chap11;

input childid bmi age gender time t1 t2 t3 sick status;

datalines;

206 15.0 59.3 0 1 1 0 0 0 0

206 15.0 63.4 0 2 0 1 0 0 0

206 14.8 66.8 0 3 0 0 1 0 0

407 18.1 25.1 0 3 0 0 1 0 1

407 17.0 17.5 0 1 1 0 0 1 1

407 16.0 21.7 0 2 0 1 0 1 1

705 15.1 70.2 1 3 0 0 1 0 1

705 15.8 62.6 1 1 1 0 0 0 1

705 15.4 66.8 1 2 0 1 0 1 1

. . . . . . . .

;
```

```
TITLE 'Model for three or more observations per person';
PROC LOGISTIC DATA=Chap11 DESCEND;
MODEL sick = BMI age t1 t2;
STRATA childid;
RUN;
```

Comment We need to identify the grouping variable. That is listed in the STRATA command. In this case, it is *childid*.

SAS Output

The LOGISTIC procedure conditional analysis	
Model information	
DataSet	WORK.MYDATA
Response variable	Sick
Number of response levels	2
Number of strata	370
Number of uninformative strata	174
Frequency uninformative	522
Model	Binary logit
Optimization technique	Newton-Raphson ridge
Number of observations read	1110
Number of observations used	1110

Comment We have 370 strata. Each stratum is identified by the *ChildId*. There are three measures for each child.

Response profile		
Ordered value	Sick	Total frequency
1	1	314
2	0	796

Comment We have 370 strata. Each stratum is identified by the *ChildId*. There are three measures for each child.

Probability modeled is sick='1'.

Comment There are 1110 = 370 × 3 cases. The 370 units were measured 3 times each. There are 314 cases when the event occurred.

Class level information			
Class	Value	Design variables	
Time	1	1	0
	2	0	1
	3	0	0

Strata summary				
Response pattern	Sick		Number of strata	Frequency
	1	0		
1	0	3	159	477
2	1	2	123	369
3	2	1	73	219
4	3	0	15	45

Comment There are four response patterns: strata with all events, strata with all nonevent, strata with one event, and strata with two events. We have 159 + 15 + 123 + 73 = 370. The frequencies 477 + 369 + 219 + 45 = 1110. There are 159 + 15 = 174 strata with no added information. There are 123 + 73 strata with information.

Newton-Raphson ridge optimization		
Without parameter scaling		
Convergence criterion (GCONV = 1E-8) satisfied.		
Model fit statistics		
Criterion	Without covariates	With covariates
AIC	430.656	428.362
SC	430.656	448.411
−2 Log L	430.656	420.362

Comment These fit statistics measure with and without the covariates. The difference tells about their significance.

Testing global null hypothesis: Beta = 0			
Test	Chi-Square	DF	Pr > ChiSq
Likelihood ratio	10.2938	4	0.0358
Score	10.1224	4	0.0384
Wald	9.9256	4	0.0417

Comment The tests (likelihood ratio, score, and Wald) provide measures for testing that covariates (BMI, age, time) are significant. These p-values suggest that they are significant.

Type 3 analysis of effects			
Effect	DF	Wald Chi-Square	Pr > ChiSq
BMI	1	0.0000	0.9959
Age	1	1.5953	0.2066
Time	2	9.7153	0.0078

Comment Time as a factor shows some significance p = 0.0078. BMI and age are not significant in this model.

Analysis of maximum likelihood estimates						
Parameter		DF	Estimate	Standard error	Wald Chi-Square	Pr > ChiSq
BMI		1	−0.00044	0.0856	0.0000	0.9959
Age		1	−0.5536	0.4383	1.5953	0.2066
Time	1	1	−4.4856	3.4613	1.6794	0.1950
Time	2	1	−2.3939	1.5103	2.5124	0.1130

Comment None of these covariates is significant (p = 0.9959, 0.2066, 0.1950, and 0.1130). The model equation though not useful in this case is:

$$\text{logit}\left(Probability_{event\ at\ time}\right) = -0.0004\text{BMI}_1 - 0.5536\text{Age}_2 - 4.4856\text{T}_1 - 2.3939\text{T}_2$$

Odds ratio estimates			
Effect	Point estimate	95% Wald confidence limits	
BMI	1.000	0.845	1.182
Age	0.575	0.244	1.357
Time 1 vs 3	0.011	<0.001	9.959
Time 2 vs 3	0.091	0.005	1.762

Comment The odds ratio will not be significant as the variable was not significant. However, the odds ratios are [0.845, 1.182] for BMI, [0.244, 1.357] for age, and the comparison of time 1 and time 2 with time 3 are [0, 9.959] and [0.005, 1.762].

11.6.2 *Fixed Effects Logistic Regression Model with More Than Two Observations Using SPSS*

SPSS Program

```
COXREG sick WITH bmi age t1 t2
/STATUS Status (1)
/STRATA=ChildID.
```

SPSS Output

Cox regression			
Case processing summary			
		N	Percent (%)
Cases available in analysis	Event[a]	588	53.0
	Censored	0	0.0
	Total	588	53.0
Cases dropped	Cases with missing values	0	0.0
	Cases with negative time	0	0.0
	Censored cases before the earliest event in a stratum	522	47.0
	Total	522	47.0
Total	1110	100.0%	

[a]Dependent ariable: Sick

Comment There are 196 informative strata each with three observations for a total of 588.

Omnibus tests of model coefficients							
−2 Log-likelihood	Overall (score)			Change from previous step			Change from previous block
	Chi-square	DF	Sig.	Chi-square	DF	Sig.	Chi-square
898.711	4.630	4	0.327	4.603	4	0.331	4.603

Comment The variables are not significant in the model ($p = 0.331$)

Omnibus tests of model coefficients	
Change from previous block	
DF	Sig.
4	0.331

Variables in the equation						
	B	SE	Wald	DF	Sig.	Exp(B)
BMI	−0.003	0.058	0.002	1	0.965	0.997
Age	0.223	0.281	0.631	1	0.427	1.250
T1	1.821	2.220	0.673	1	0.412	6.176
T2	0.990	0.967	1.048	1	0.306	2.692

[a]Beginning block number 1. Method = Enter

Comment logit($Probability_{event\ at\ time}$) = $-0.003BMI_1 + 0.223Age_2 + 1.821T_1 + 0.990T_2$. Neither BMI, age, nor time is significant. We write out the model for clarity.

Covariate means	
	Mean
BMI	15.368
Age	42.058
T1	0.333
T2	0.333

Case processing summary			
Unweighted cases[a]		N	Percent
Selected cases	Included in analysis	134	100.0
	Missing cases	0	0.0
	Total	134	100.0
Unselected cases		0	0.0
Total		134	100.0

[a]If weight is in effect, see the classification table for the total number of cases

11.6.3 *Fixed Effects Logistic Regression Model with More Than Two Observations Using R*

R Program

```
> data1$time.f <- factor(data1$time)
> clogit.out=clogit(formula = sick ~ 0 + bmi + age +
relevel(time.f, ref=3) + strata(childid), data = data1)
> summary(clogit.out)
Call:
coxph(formula = Surv(rep(1, 1110L), sick) ~ 0 + bmi + age +
relevel(time.f,
    ref = 3) + strata(childid), data = data1, method = "exact")
```

Comment We use clogit for conditional logit models.

R Output

```
Deviance Residuals:
  n= 1110, number of events= 314
          coef         exp(coef)   se(coef)     z           Pr(>|z|)
BMI     -0.0004359  0.9995642  0.0856364  -0.005      0.996
age     -0.5535719  0.5748927  0.4382821  -1.263      0.207
relevel(time.f, ref = 3)1 -4.4856334  0.0112697  3.4613209
-1.296    0.195
relevel(time.f, ref = 3)2 -2.3938713  0.0912756  1.5102823
-1.585         0.113
```

Comment The variables are not significant in the model. You are given the coefficient (coef); the exponential of (coef), i.e., e^{coeff}; and the standard errors. The model though not significant (for clarity) is:

$$\text{logit}\left(Probability_{event\ at\ time}\right) = -0.0004\text{BMI}_1 - 0.5536\text{Age}_2 - 4.4856\text{T}_1 - 2.3939\text{T}_2$$

```
                exp(coef)     exp(-coef)   lower .95     upper .95
bmi             0.99956       1.000          8.451e-01     1.182
age             0.57489       1.739          2.435e-01     1.357
relevel(time.f, ref = 3)1   0.01127  88.733   1.275e-05     9.959
relevel(time.f, ref = 3)2   0.0912   10.956   4.729e-03     1.762
```

Comment If we were to take exp.(−0.0004359) = 0.999564. The 95% confidence interval is [$8.451 \times 10^{-1,}$ 1.182].

```
Rsquare= 0.009   (max possible= 0.322)
Likelihood ratio test= 10.29 on 4 df,   p=0.03576
Wald test            = 9.93 on 4 df,    p=0.0417
Score (logrank) test = 10.12 on 4 df,   p=0.03842
```

Comment The likelihood ratio test, Wald test, and logrank test do not support significance for the simultaneous effect of the covariates.

11.6.4 Fixed Effects Logistic Regression Model with More Than Two Observations Using STATA

STATA

```
clogit sick bmi age t1 t2, group(childid)
note: multiple positive outcomes within groups encountered.
note: 174 groups (522 obs) omitted because of all positive or
      all negative outcomes.
Iteration 0:  Log-likelihood = -211.47657
Iteration 3:  Log-likelihood = -210.18109
Conditional (fixed effects) logistic regression      Number of obs = 588
                          LR chi2(4)     =  10.29
                          Prob > chi2    = 0.0358
Log likelihood = -210.18109                        Pseudo R2   = 0.0239

 Sick | Coefficient  Std. err.   z     P>|z|    [95% conf. interval]
BMI  |  -.0004359  .0856364  -0.01  0.996    -.1682801    .1674084
Age  |  -.5535719  .4382821  -1.26  0.207    -1.412589    .3054451
 t1  |  -4.485633 3.461321   -1.30  0.195   -11.2697     2.298431
 t2  |  -2.393871 1.510282   -1.59  0.113    -5.35397     .5662277
```

Comment logit($Probability_{event\ at\ time}$) = $-0.0004BMI_1 + 0.5536Age_2 - 0.496T_1 - 2.394T_2$. Neither BMI, age, nor time is significant. We write out the model for clarity.

11.7 Conclusions

Some researchers prefer fixed effects models because they are less likely to have omitted variable bias (Allison, 2005). In cases where the within-person variation is small relative to the between-person variation, the standard errors of the fixed effects coefficients may be too large to accept as an adequate approach. By using each individual as his or her own control, fixed effects regression methods provide a relatively easy and effective way to control for time-independent variables that cannot be measured. However, analyzing the data using the fixed effects logistic regression model allows one to control for covariates that have not been measured, we can make causal inferences from non-experimental data, and we can account for covariates that cannot be measured.

11.8 Related Examples

To help the reader expand the thought process of situations where the fixed effects logistic regression model may be useful, we refer the reader to the National Longitudinal Surveys (NLS). NLS is a set of surveys that were designed to gather information at successive points in time on the labor market and other significant life events of several groups of men and women. The interviews began in 1966 for the NLS older men, a group of 5020 men ages 45–59. Older men were near retirement and needing to think about the timing and extent of their labor force and deciding to stop. Data collection focused on topics such as work and nonwork experiences, retirement planning, health conditions, insurance coverage, and the approach to time spent with their leisure activities. The survey also tracked labor market decisions such as middle-aged job changes, retirement expectations and experiences, and reentry to the labor market after initial retirement. Interviews with this cohort ceased in 1981. In 1990, information was collected from respondents and widows or other next of kin of deceased sample members. The data a.\lso includes cause of death information collected from state vital records departments in 1990.

http://www.bls.gov/nls/oldyoungmen.htm. There are binary responses such that one may wish to model. The types of information gathered in survey are work experience, including retirement, education, household composition, family background, marital status and marital transitions, income and assets, health, and attitudes.

References

Agresti, A. (2007). *An introduction to categorical data analysis*. Wiley.

Allison, P. D. (2005). *Fixed effects regression methods for longitudinal data using SAS*. SAS Institute Inc.

Bhargava, A. (1994). Modelling the health of Filipino children. *Journal of the Royal Statistical Society, Series A, 157*(3), 417–432.

Harris, P., Brennan, J., Martin, J., Gould, D., Bakran, A., Smith, G. G., Buth, J., Gevers, E., & White, D. (1999). Longitudinal aneurysm shrinkage following endovascular aortic aneurysm repair: A source of intermediate and late complications. *Journal of Endovascular Surgery, 6*(1), 11–16.

Kohler, U., & Kreuter, F. (2012). *Data analysis using stata* (2nd ed., p. 245).

Lai, T. L., & Small, D. (2007). Marginal regression analysis of longitudinal data with time-dependent covariates: A generalized method of moments approach. *Journal of the Royal Statistical Society: Series B (Statistical Methodology), 69*(1), 79–99.

Sobel, M. E. (2000). Causal inference in the social sciences. *Journal of the American Statistical Association, 95*(450), 647–651.

Wooldridge, J. M. (2002). *Econometric analysis of cross section and panel data*. The MIT Press.

Part IV
Analyzing Correlated Data Through the Joint Modeling of Mean and Variance

Chapter 12
Heteroscedastic Logistic Regression Model

12.1 Motivating Example

There is increased interest in modeling correlated binary data. The correlation presents some natural challenges over the complete independent observations situation. In the fit of a logistic regression model, we can never include all the predictors that affect the binary response. As such, there will always be some unobserved unmeasurable factors. As these are unmeasurable and unobservable, it is customary to account for them through a random term. However, the omission of relevant covariates leads to increased unobserved heterogeneity, and as such, it affects the regression coefficients of the remaining regressor as it pertains to significance (Cramer, 2006). Cramer found through a simulation that omitting a relevant variable lead to severe misspecification of the disturbance. Further, he pointed out that the unexplained variation is included in a disturbance term which is treated as a random variable. In so doing, we want to concentrate on the variance of this random disturbance, which without loss of generality is assumed to be of zero mean. The problem is that if the variance of the random effects is not constant for all subpopulations found in our mean model, then we have heterogeneity. It is an established fact as a rule logistic regression is quite robust if the distribution of the error term is incorrect. Such a phenomenon led us to concur that modeling both the mean and the variance simultaneously is worth exploring.

The joint modeling of the mean and dispersion is not necessarily new. In the past, we have used constant dispersion, but now we want to have nonconstant dispersion as it seems more practical. Constant dispersion models have indeed in many ways been addressed in this text in Chap. 4 when we used the overdispersed logistic regression model. In particular, we used the beta-binomial model. In such cases, the intraclass correlation was of interest. That is unlike the GEE logistic regression model (Chap. 6), which is suitable for cases when there is no real interest in the dispersion or the intraclass correlation. Methods involved in estimating the

J. R. Wilson et al., *Modeling Binary Correlated Responses*, ICSA Book Series in Statistics, https://doi.org/10.1007/978-3-031-62427-8_12

parameters in the mean sub-model and dispersion sub-model include the extended beta-binomial, the quasi-likelihood and other moment methods, the extended quasi-likelihood, the Gaussian likelihood, and the quadratic estimating equations (Paul & Islam, 1998).

We revisit the simulated Hospital, Doctor, Patient (HDP) dataset. This dataset has a three-level, hierarchical structure with patients nested within doctors, and doctors nested within hospitals. The purpose of the simulated data is to create a rich dataset that can be used to show a variety of analytic techniques. We concentrate on age, length of stay, and doctor's experience as it pertains to cancer remission. The study was meant to be a large study of lung cancer outcomes across multiple doctors and sites. However, we do not believe that age, length of stay, and doctor's experience are enough to explain cancer remission. The other factors not observed or measured are part of the random effects. These random effects are assumed to have a mean of zero and an unknown variance and more often than not normally distributed. We used age, length of stay, and doctor's experience to model the unobserved variation. We use a dispersion sub-model to investigate the variance as we assume they are related to some known factors. In our demonstration, we use age, length of stay, and doctor's experience but could have used other covariates not considered in the mean sub-model. For a complete discussion and theoretical derivation of the joint modeling of the mean and dispersion, we refer the interested reader to Nelder and Lee (1992; 2002).

12.2 Definitions and Notations

Joint modeling refers to the simultaneous modeling of the response associated with the mean and the response associated with the dispersion.

The *mean sub-model* is the portion of the joint model that addresses the mean of the response, including distributional assumptions of the responses, the predictors of the mean, and a possible link function of the mean and the covariates.

The *dispersion sub-model* is the portion of the joint model that addresses the response variation. It includes the distributional assumptions, the predictors of the variance, and a possible link function of the variance and the covariates.

Random effects (Chap. 9) are the unobservable differential effects among clusters. They are useful in avoiding erroneous conclusions. They are used to estimate population variance and include sampling variation. They consist of a sample of items from a large population that have varying effects on the response. They are therefore unobservable but believed to belong to a population with a certain mean and variance. They are used to address clustering, spatial correlation, and other forms of dependence among outcomes and are usually assumed to be normally distributed. Our interest is in their variance. If the variance is estimated to be different from zero, we assume that there are differential effects.

12.3 Exploratory Analyses

The HDP data are analyzed in Chap. 10 using logistic regression with random intercepts and random slopes to model the variability among patients and among doctors. A subset of that dataset is given in Table 12.1.

We revisit these data but now account for the heterogeneity through a sub-model. Recall there are 8525 patients in the dataset with 407 doctors and 85 hospitals. We have an interest in assessing the impact of certain covariates on the probability of remission but want to account for the heterogeneity that may be presently associated across subpopulations. If we were to fit the logistic regression model, then we will have 6004 in remission (=0) and 2521 not in cancer remission (=1) with age, length of stay, and doctor's experience as covariates. The likelihood ratio is 322.13 with three degrees of freedom, $p < 0.0001$. We find that for the standard mean sub-model, we obtained the results in Table 12.2. Hosmer and Lemeshow's statistic ($p = 0.0414$) showed that the model is not a good fit.

We cannot really proceed with this so-called fitted model:

$$logit\ \hat{p} = -0.288 - 0.021 Age - 0.184 LOS + 0.084 Experience$$

since the model is not a good fit. However, we took the deviance residuals and fitted with covariates age, length of stay, and doctor's experience. We obtain the results in Table 12.3. The covariates, age, and doctor's experience seem to be important in addressing the heterogeneity. However, though it is not necessarily a scientific approach, we examine some graphical explorations as they are necessary in understanding heterogeneity.

A graph of the predicted probabilities versus age shows that as age increases the probability of remission decreases in the figures that follow. Also predicted probability versus experience or length of stay also has definite patterns. It is clear that heterogeneity is present.

Table 12.1 Subset of HDP dataset

Remission	Age	Length of stay	Experience	DID
0	64.96824	6	25	1
0	53.91714	6	25	1
0	53.3473	5	25	1
0	41.36804	5	25	1
0	46.80042	6	25	1
0	51.92936	5	25	1
0	53.82926	4	25	1
0	46.56223	5	25	1
0	54.38936	6	25	1
.	.	.	.	.
.	.	.	.	.

Table 12.2 Analysis of maximum likelihood estimates

	Standard			Wald	
Parameter	DF	Estimate	Error	Chi-Square	Pr > ChiSq
Intercept	1	−0.2882	0.2254	1.6348	0.2010
Age	1	−0.0213	0.00434	23.9521	<0.0001
Length of stay	1	−0.1842	0.0260	50.1282	<0.0001
Experience	1	0.0838	0.00605	192.0264	<0.0001

Table 12.3 Parameter estimates for deviance

	Parameter		Standard		
Variable	DF	Estimate	Error	t-value	Pr > |t|
Age	1	−0.00314	0.00152	−2.07	0.0388
Length of stay	1	−0.02139	0.01224	−1.75	0.0806
Experience	1	0.00874	0.00256	3.41	0.0007

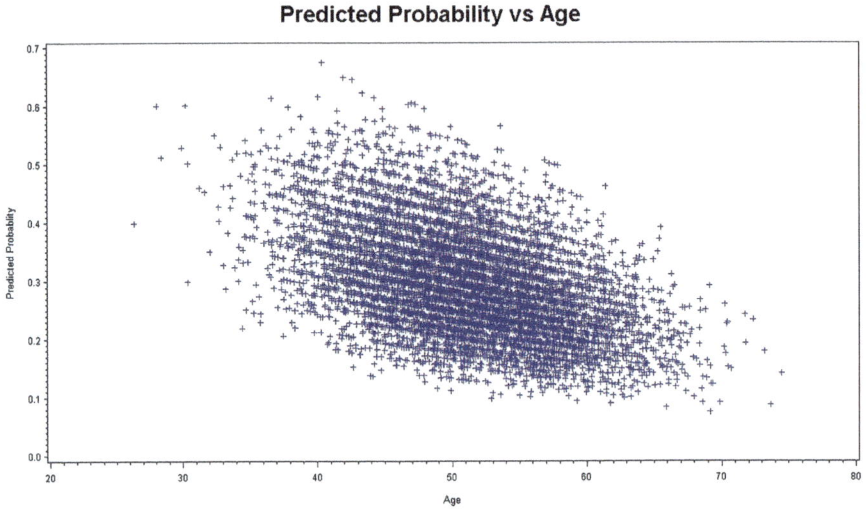

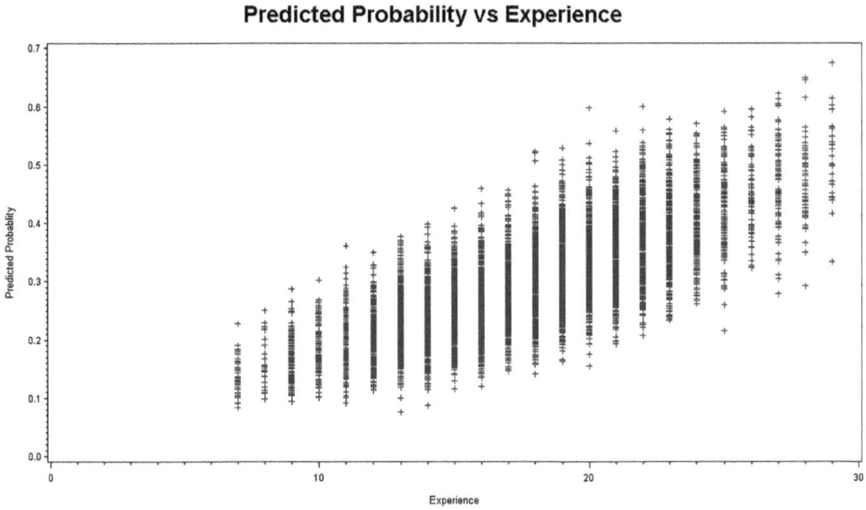

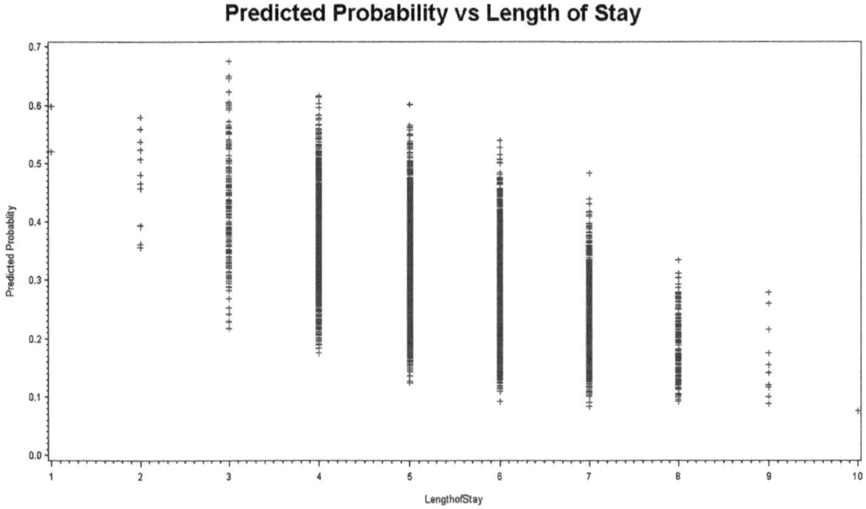

12.3.1 Dispersion Sub-model

In his well-known paper, Professor Efron introduces the idea of joint modeling, where both means and variances are allowed to depend on observed covariates (Efron, 1986). Prior, we normally relied on the one-parameter exponential family, where the mean and variance are related. However, in the normal regression models, the variance is not related to the mean. Several researchers have considered

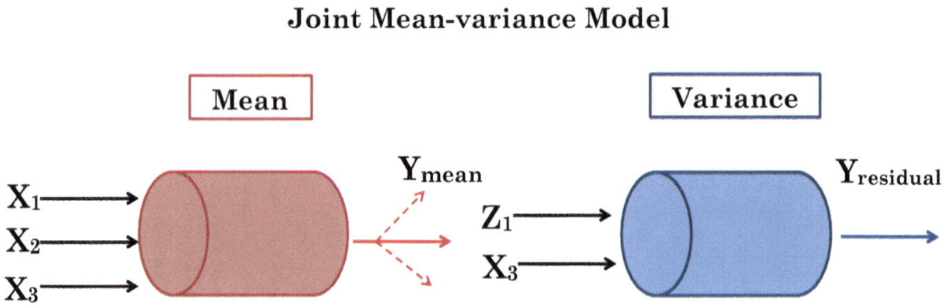

Fig. 12.1 Joint mean-variance model

dispersion modeling for normal data (Aitkin, 1987; Carroll & Rupert, 1987; Davidian & Carroll, 1987, 1988). Smyth (1989) shows that similar methods are used for a certain class of non-normal generalized linear models. A similar structure using the residuals obtained for the mean sub-model as the responses fit in the so-called dispersion sub-model. Thus, the extension allowed the variance to be modeled through the deviance d_i from the mean sub-model in the same manner as the responses were modeled in the original mean sub-model. There are three components: random, systematic, and link. The systematic component consists of either all, some, or none of the factors from the mean sub-model or may include some new factors. This gives rise to the joint modeling of the mean and variance (Lee et al., 2006), as depicted in Fig. 12.1.

12.4 Statistical Model

It seems to be an established fact that correct modeling of the dispersion is necessary (Wu & Li, 2012). There is a loss in efficiency in using constant dispersion models when there is significant heterogeneity. Other researchers have used the double generalized linear models to look at the joint modeling of the mean and dispersion modeling (Smyth & Verbyla, 1999). The joint modeling of mean and dispersion consists of two sub-models, each following a generalized linear model, for example, Table 12.4.

Consider the response, whether or not a person's cancer is in remission as a Bernoulli distribution with covariates age of patient, length of stay, and doctor's experience.

- When the joint sub-model is fitted, the deviance component from the mean sub-model becomes the response for the dispersion sub-model.
- The covariate in the dispersion sub-model, Table 12.4, is the length of stay.
- We use the fit values to estimate the variance of the response in the mean sub-model thereby providing useful weights to fit that model.
- A log link is chosen for the dispersion sub-model.

Table 12.4 Mean and dispersion sub-models of the joint modeling

Mean sub-model	Dispersion sub-model
$\text{Remission}_i \sim \text{Bernoulli}\ (p_i, p_i(1-p_i))$	$d_i \sim \mathcal{D}_d(\phi_i, V_{di}(\phi_i))$
$\eta_i = \beta_0 + \beta_1 Age + \beta_2 LOS + \beta_4 Experience$	$\eta_{di} = \gamma_0 + \gamma_1 Age + \gamma_2 LOS + \gamma_3 Experience$
$\eta_i = logit\ (p_i)$	$\eta_{di} = \log \phi_i$

- We continue such a process for four or five cycles (Nelder & Lee, 1998).
- We have a model consisting of two interlinked GLMs, one for the mean and one for the dispersion (Nelder & Lee, 1991).
- Weights used in the mean sub-model are calculated using the results of the dispersion sub-model.
- Thus, the two models are connected through parameters in one model calculated from the other.
- There are two important characteristics of this model.
  - First, the expected value of the deviance components does not equal the parameter, so there is a small bias.
  - Second, the assumed distribution of the deviance is not necessarily a gamma (Nelder & Lee, 1998). The choice of the link function for the dispersion sub-model is not necessarily as key a component.
- However, in many studies, the modeling of the dispersion will be sufficient to identify and account for the sources of variability. Smyth and Verba used the chi-square approximation for the deviance as is the case when we use PROC QLIM in SAS to fit the joint modeling of the mean and dispersion.
  Table 12.4 presents a joint generalized linear model consisting of three components for the mean sub-model and three components for the dispersion sub-model, as it pertains to the Medicare data. The d_i represents the deviance from the mean sub-model with mean and variance.

12.4.1 *Joint Modeling*

In fact, the modeling of correlated binomial data is a fit through a mean model if the interest is only on the mean and the dispersion is considered a nuisance parameter. However, if the intraclass correlation is of interest, then it is necessary to use a joint modeling of the mean and the dispersion (Efron, 1986) (one of the first to model both the mean and the variance). The dispersion sub-model allows extra parameters to model the variance independent of the mean, thus allowing covariates to be included in both the mean and variance sub-models. In this chapter, we present sub-models that analyze simultaneously the mean and the dispersion. The two sub-models are based on the generalized linear model.

The theory of generalized linear models (Dobson, 1990; McCullagh & Nelder, 1989; Nelder & Wedderburn, 1972) provided an extension to linear models as it allows the response to have a distribution other than normal and the relation between the mean and the covariates to be linked in other ways than the identity link. In particular, a generalized linear model consists of three components (as it concentrates on modeling the mean of the response distribution): the random component, in which the distribution $\mathcal{D}$ of the response is known; the systematic component, which tells about the combination based on the covariates X_1, X_2, ...X_p; and the link component, which tells the relationship g between the combination of covariates and the response mean μ_i. In summary, the response Y_i is distributed with mean μ_i with a covariance σ_i^2 and distribution $\mathcal{D}$, which belongs to the exponentia family, such that $g(\mu_i) = f(X_1, X_2, \ldots\ldots X_p)$. Generalized linear models model responses are not normally distributed (McCullagh & Nelder, 1989). They are more general than the linear model methods in that they allow modeling the mean based on the assumption that certain covariates are approximately linear. However, it is just as crucial to model the variance when there is heterogeneity. It is a fact that efficient estimation of mean parameters in regression with covariates depends on correctly modeling the dispersion (Smyth & Verbyla, 1999). The loss of efficiency is great if we ignore heterogeneity when it is present. Modeling of the dispersion is also necessary to obtain correct standard errors and confidence intervals (Carroll & Rupert, 1987, 1988; Smyth, 1989).

While the works of Efron (1986) introduce the joint modeling of the mean and dispersion through likelihood techniques, Pregibon (1984) introduces the joint modeling of the mean and dispersion through the use of the three components of the generalized linear model for both the mean and dispersion. Smyth (1989) also contributes to the joint modeling research. Efron's approach made use of the double exponential family through the addition of a parameter to the one-parameter exponential family. Lalonde et al. (2014) looked at hierarchical joint models. The analysis of joint modeling of both the mean and the dispersion, each with its own set of covariates is appropriate when the regression relationship is being used to study any effect of covariates on both the mean and variance of the responses. Joint modeling is also an appropriate approach when there is the main interest in identifying the effects of covariates on the variance of the responses, as an initial mean sub-model is often necessary when modeling dispersion. While extended quasi-likelihood and generalized extended quasi-likelihood models include additional components to account for modeling the dispersion. They are both special cases of joint generalized linear models. They specify the form of the mean–variance relationship for dispersion sub-model include no covariate, thus implicitly defining a systematic component with only a constant term.

The heteroscedastic logistic model when fitted using the hetero option with PROC QLIM in SAS assumed that you are using a log link with the overdispersion sub-model with a normalizing constant. The two models (mean sub-model and dispersion sub-model) are interlinked as shown in Fig. 12.2 (Nelder & Lee, 1998). The

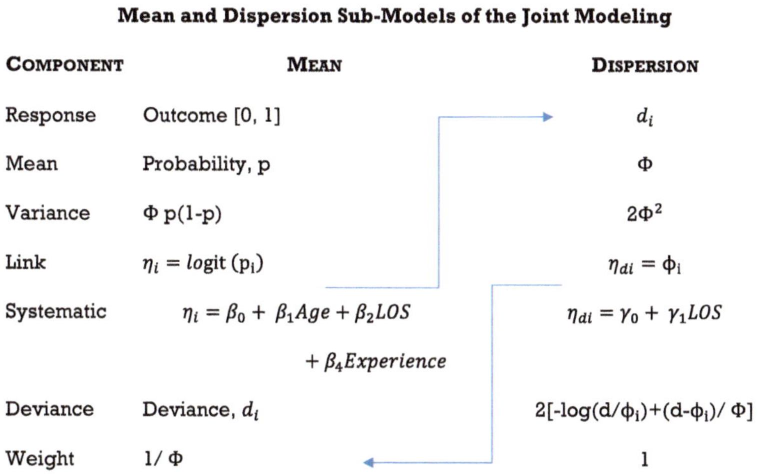

Fig. 12.2 Mean and dispersion sub-models of the joint modeling

process of fitting these sub-models works as follows. We first fit the mean sub-model. The deviance from the fit of the mean sub-model with its covariates is then used as the responses in the dispersion sub-model. Once we fit the dispersion sub-model, we used the fitted values as measures of dispersion become the weights for the mean sub-model and the process is repeated. We learned from Nelder and Lee (1998) and we concur that this takes about 4–5 cycles.

12.5 Analysis of Data

12.5.1 Heteroscedastic Logistic Regression Model

We revisit the HDP data. In so doing, we present the joint modeling of the mean and dispersion. We had a reason to believe that the variance may be influenced by sources related to the length of stay (LOS). Methods for modeling overdispersed data are presented through the joint modeling of mean and variance. These methods are of two kinds: a likelihood approach and a method-of-moments approach. Likelihood methods require knowledge of the distribution. The likelihood method facilitates computation of maximum likelihood estimates, which can be obtained through the same algorithm as that of weighted least squares, while the quasi-likelihood or moment approaches (does not require knowledge of the distribution) seem to be appropriate when severe overdispersion may be present. We fitted the joint model using SAS and R.

SAS Program

```
PROC QLIM DATA=mydata;
MODEL biRadmit=Age LOS Experience/ DISCRETE(D=LOGIT);
HETERO biRadmit ~ Age LOS Experience;
RUN;
```

Comment The QLIM (qualitative and limited dependent variable model) procedure can be used to analyze the joint mean and dispersion sub-model. The QLIM procedure mainly uses the maximum likelihood (ML) method for the sub-model. The structural parameters are estimated in the second stage using the least squares method (The QLIM Procedure in SAS manual). The heteroscedastic logistic regression model has its dispersion sub-model estimated using the HETERO statement. In the dispersion sub-model age, length of stay, and doctor's experience are believed to have an impact on the variance. In our analysis, the variance can be specified as

$$\mathrm{var}\left(\mathrm{d_i}\right) = \sigma^2 \exp\left(\gamma_1 \mathrm{LOS} + \gamma_2 \mathrm{Age} + \gamma_3 \mathrm{Experience}\right)$$

where σ^2 is the variance parameter and γ_1, $\gamma_{2,}$ and γ_3 are coefficients for the covariates in the dispersion sub-model. The HETERO statement specifies the covariates (age, length of stay, and doctor's experience) believed to influence the dispersion and the form of that relationship. It assumes that the random component in the dispersion sub-model is normal with mean zero and variance σ^2.

SAS Output

Discrete response profile of remission			
Index	Value	Frequency	Percent
1	0	6004	70.43
2	1	2521	29.57

Comment There were 8525 observations with 2521 patients in remission of cancer and 6004 who did not.

Model fit summary	
Number of endogenous variables	1
Endogenous variable	Remission
Number of observations	8525
Log likelihood	−5006
Maximum absolute gradient	0.0001156
Number of iterations	46
Optimization method	Quasi-Newton
AIC	10,027
Schwarz criterion	10,076

Comment The endogenous variable is our output variable. A likelihood approach is used to tell if the model is a good fit. The log-likelihood is −5006, so -2log-likelihood is 10,012. AIC and Schwarz criterion have values 10,027 and 10,076, respectively.

Goodness-of-fit measures		
Measure	Value	Formula
Likelihood ratio (R)	339.85	2 * (LogL - LogL0)
Upper bound of R (U)	10,353	- 2 * LogL0
Aldrich-nelson	0.0383	R/(R + N)
Cragg-Uhler 1	0.0391	1 - exp (-R/N)
Cragg-Uhler 2	0.0556	(1-exp(-R/N))/(1-exp(-U/N))
Estrella	0.0397	1 - (1-R/U)^(U/N)
Adjusted Estrella	0.0381	1 - ((LogL-K)/LogL0)^(-2/N*LogL0)
McFadden's LRI	0.0328	R/U
Veall-Zimmermann	0.0699	(R * (U + N))/(U * (R + N))
McKelvey-Zavoina	0.0347	
N = # of observations, K = # of regressors		

Comment There are several goodness-of-fit measures given. These measures have received mixed reviews in the literature. SAS PROC QLIM handout reveals that all measures except McKelvey-Zavoina's definition are based on the log-likelihood function value (see SAS Manual on PROC QLIM). The likelihood ratio test statistic has chi-square distribution conditional on the null hypothesis that all slope coefficients are zero. In this example, the likelihood ratio statistic is used to test the hypothesis that coefficients age, length of stay, and doctor's experience are all equal to zero.

Parameter estimates					
Parameter	DF	Estimate	Standard error	t value	Approx Pr > |t|
Intercept	1	−0.395745	0.145357	−2.72	0.0065
Age	1	0.000397	0.006027	0.07	0.9475
LOS	1	−0.131164	0.090128	−1.46	0.1456
Experience	1	0.032680	0.017840	1.83	0.0670
_H.Age	1	−0.054733	0.022064	−2.48	0.0131
_H.Los	1	0.075753	0.139593	0.54	0.5874
_H.Experience	1	0.078591	0.028942	2.72	0.0066

Comment The mean sub-model is

$$\text{logit}p = -0.396 + 0.0003Age - 0.131LOS + 0.033Experience$$

The parameter estimates in the dispersion sub-model for heteroscedasticity are listed as H_age, H_LOS, and H_experience. The HETERO statement specifies variables that are related to the heteroscedasticity of the residuals and the way these variables are used to model the error variance. The heteroscedastic regression model supported by PROC QLIM is $\log \sigma_i^2 = -0.055 Age + 0.076 LOS + 0.079 Experience$. When the LINK = option is not specified, PROC QLIM assumes the exponential link function, which was the case here.

12.5.2 Standard Logistic Regression Model

SAS Program

```
PROC QLIM DATA=mydata
MODEL biRadmit=Age LOS Experience/ DISCRETE(D=LOGIT)
RUN;
```

SAS Output

Discrete response profile of remission			
Index	Value	Frequency	Percent
1	0	6004	70.43
2	1	2521	29.57

Comment There are 29.57% or 2512 patients with cancer in remission.

Model fit summary	
Number of endogenous variables	1
Endogenous variable	Remission
Number of observations	8525
Log likelihood	−5015
Maximum absolute gradient	0.00639
Number of iterations	14
Optimization method	Quasi-Newton
AIC	10,039
Schwarz criterion	10,067

Comment The endogenous variable is cancer in remission versus it is not. The method used to obtain parameter estimates is the Quasi-Newton.

Goodness-of-fit measures		
Measure	Value	Formula
Likelihood ratio (R)	322.13	2 * (LogL - LogL0)
Upper bound of R (U)	10,353	- 2 * LogL0
Aldrich-nelson	0.0364	R/(R + N)
Cragg-Uhler 1	0.0371	1 - exp (-R/N)
Cragg-Uhler 2	0.0527	(1-exp (-R/N))/(1-exp(-U/N))
Estrella	0.0377	1 - (1-R/U)^(U/N)
Adjusted Estrella	0.0367	1 - ((LogL-K)/LogL0)^(-2/N*LogL0)
McFadden's LRI	0.0311	R/U
Veall-Zimmermann	0.0664	(R * (U + N))/(U * (R + N))
McKelvey-Zavoina	0.1608	
N = # of observations, K = # of regressors		

Comment There are goodness-of-fit measures for the model. We found that Cragg-Uhler to be most useful.

Parameter estimates					
Parameter	DF	Estimate	Standard error	t value	Approx Pr > |t|
Intercept	1	−0.288241	0.225428	−1.28	0.2010
Age	1	−0.021259	0.004343	−4.89	<0.0001
Length of stay	1	−0.184241	0.026023	−7.08	<0.0001
Experience	1	0.083797	0.006047	13.86	<0.0001

Comment The mean sub-model is for the standard logistic regression model is

$$\text{logit}p = -0.289 - 0.021Age - 0.184LOS + 0.084Experience$$

The covariates age, length of stay, and experience are significant. However, this was not the case in heteroscedastic logistic regression model.

12.5.3 Model Comparisons Mean Sub-model Versus Joint Modeling

A comparison of the impact of the covariates as they exist in the mean model (standard logistic regression model) versus a mean and dispersion sub-model (heteroscedastic logistic regression model) is made. Neither age, length of stay, nor doctor's years of experience seem to be significant when the extra variation is modeled (Table 12.5). The covariates age, length of stay, and experience are significant.

Table 12.5 Mean sub-model covariates in the mean model versus in the joint modeling

	Mean and dispersion submodels	Mean submodel
Age	+ sign with $p = 0.9475$	– sign with $p < 0.0001$
Length of stay	– sign with $p = 0.1456$	– sign with $p < 0.0001$
Experience	+ sign with $p = 0.0670$	+ sign with $p < 0.0001$

However, this is not significant when the extra variation is modeled. The sign of the covariate *Age* (though insignificant) was reversed.

12.6 Conclusions

A heteroscedastic logistic regression model is presented in which the data are analyzed with a mean-dispersion relationship in the dispersion sub-models while considering fixed and random effects. In addition, the model allows for covariates to be included in both the mean and dispersion sub-models. While the pseudo-likelihood model is applicable for response distributions belonging to the exponential family, its systematic component is approximated by restricting to a first-order normal random variable and only allows for a constant dispersion correction and as such cannot include covariates in the dispersion sub-model. Though the double-extended quasi-likelihood model is applicable for any response with random effects from distributions belonging to the exponential family and does allow dispersion sub-models with covariates, it imposes a specific mean-variance relationship for both dispersion sub-models.

12.7 Related Examples

Many researchers have studied issues related to immigrant's English proficiency. Gender, educational level, and age at migration can affect English proficiency (Jasso & Rosenzweig, 1986). Race can also be considered as a predictor variable since immigrants from "Romance-language" countries may learn English better than immigrants from Asian countries (Loo, 1985). For immigrant children, it is suggested that parents' education level is highly related to student performance (Abedi et al., 2003). Also, immigrants with higher occupational accomplishments are more proficient in English. Larger household size is associated with lower proficiency. LEP students' percentage in a class and class size may also influence English proficiency (Abedi, 2004). Therefore, students' gender, students' race, mother's employment status, father's employment status, race of mother, race of father, students' disability status, number of siblings in the household, total number in household, mother's education level, father's education level, average prestige score for mother's occupation, average prestige score for father's occupation, poverty status, percent of minority in class, teacher's age, percent of LEP students in class, teacher's gender, and teacher's education level may be key factors in modeling success in proficiency. Data from Early Childhood Longitudinal Studies-Kindergarten Class of 1998–1999 from the National Center for Education Statistics, the US Department of Education can be considered. A total of 21,260 children was sampled across the United States. The data are longitudinal from the fall of 1998 through fifth grade. We chose a subset of the data from fall 1998 to spring 2000, including children who do not speak English language at home to predict factors affecting their English proficiency. In the fall of 1998, 2005 students took the exam and 867 passed. In spring 1999, 1066 students took the exam and 390 passed. In the fall of 1999, 177 students took the exam and 41 passed. In spring 2000, 522 students took the exam and 298 passed; our data shows that many students who did not take the exam in fall 1999 took the exam in spring 2000. The data are unbalanced longitudinal in that once a student passes the exam, he or she will not take the exam again. Unlike traditional longitudinal data, it repeated measuring one subject over time. The data have a hierarchical structure. It was collected on students clustered within classrooms, and classrooms were sampled within schools. The first level is the student; the second level is classroom; and the third level is school.

12.7.1 Logistic Predicted

Remission	Age	Length of stay	Experience	DID	predicted	deviance_resid
0	47.24938	5	14	2	0.358571	−0.9423983
1	43.7356	5	14	2	0.354057	1.44103978
1	53.14721	7	14	2	0.487	1.19957605
1	49.11262	5	14	2	0.360975	1.42754705
0	64.52788	4	14	2	0.324528	−0.88582607
0	47.63018	5	14	2	0.359062	−0.94321016
0	66.36314	6	14	2	0.44368	−1.08297036
1	50.98166	7	14	2	0.48397	1.204768
0	49.08775	4	14	2	0.305863	−0.85450095
1	45.9149	5	19	3	0.816431	0.63688785
0	51.0809	4	19	3	0.28661	−0.82185999
1	50.92295	5	19	3	0.526458	1.13276922
0	49.75095	6	19	3	0.802897	−1.80223616
1	56.18753	8	19	3	0.827903	0.61458883
1	47.53297	5	19	3	0.739699	0.77654541
0	53.50774	4	18	4	0.290181	−0.82794286
0	49.5336	6	18	4	0.19933	−0.66679371
0	56.47173	4	18	4	0.187851	−0.64509054
0	49.46599	6	18	4	0.201412	−0.67068601
0	49.68009	6	18	4	0.194876	−0.65842054

Remission	Age	Length of stay	Experience	DID	predicted	deviance_resid
1	44.61022	5	18	4	0.546204	1.09978399
1	58.08923	6	18	4	0.045894	2.48250989
0	51.88174	6	18	4	0.136853	−0.54253126
0	52.8699	6	18	4	0.115929	−0.49642406
1	40.10036	5	18	4	0.741143	0.77403139
1	51.45639	3	18	4	0.532321	1.1229503
0	65.61566	7	18	4	0.005997	−0.10968328
1	45.40815	6	18	4	0.354852	1.43948315
0	60.88663	7	18	4	0.014748	−0.17238389
0	53.94108	5	18	4	0.166925	−0.60437049

References

Abedi, J. (2004). The no child left behind act and English language learners: Assessment and accountability issues. *Educational Researcher, 33*, 1.

Abedi, J., Courtney, M., & Leon, S. (2003). *Research-supported accommodation for English language learners in NAEP* (CSE Tech. Rep. No. 586).

Aitkin, M. (1987). Modelling variance heterogeneity in normal regression using GLIM. *Journal of the Royal Statistical Society: Series C. Applied Statistics, 36*(3), 332–339.

Carroll, R. J., & Ruppert, D. (1987). Diagnostics and robust estimation when transforming the response and the regression model. *Technometrics, 29*(3), 287–299.

Carroll, R. J., & Ruppert, D. (1988). *Transformation and weighting in regression*. Chapman and Hall.

Cramer, J. S. (2006). Robustness of logit analysis: *Unobserved heterogeneity and misspecified disturbances* (Discussion Paper 2006/07). Amsterdam School of Economics Department of Quantitative Economics UvA Econometrics.

Davidian, M., & Carroll, R. J. (1987). Variance function estimation. *Journal ofAmerican Statistical Association, 82*(400), 1079–1091.

Dobson, A. J. (1990). *An introduction to generalized linear models*. Chapman and Hall.

Efron, B. E. (1986). Double exponential families and their use in generalized linear regression. *Journal of the American Statistical Association, 81*(395), 709–721.

Jasso, G., & Rosenzweig, M. R. (1986). What's in a name? Country of origin influences on the earning of immigrants in the United States. *Research in Human Capital and Development, 2*(4), 75–106.

Lalonde, T. L., Wilson, J. R., & Yin, J. (2014). GMM logistic regression models for longitudinal data with time-dependent covariates and extended classifications. *Statistics in Medicine, 33*(27), 4756–4769.

Lee, Y., Nelder, J. A., & Pawitan, Y. (2006). *Generalized linear models with random effects: Unified analysis via H-likelihood*. Chapman and Hall/CRC Ulva Monographs on Statistics and Applied Probability.

Loo, C. M. (1985). Biliterate ballot controversy: Language acquisition and cultural shift among immigrants. *International Migration Review, 19*, 493–515.

McCullagh, P., & Nelder, J. A. (1989). *Generalized linear models* (2nd ed.). Chapman and Hall/CRC Monographs on Statistics and Applied Probability.

Nelder, J. A., & Lee, Y. (1991). Generalized linear models for the analysis of taguchi-type experiments. *Applied Stochastic Models in and Data Analysis, 7*(1), 107–120.

Nelder, J. A., & Lee, Y. (1992). Likelihood, quasi-likelihood and pseudo likelihood: some comparisons. *Journal of the Royal Statistical Society Series B: Statistical Methodology, 54*(1), 273–284.

Nelder, J. A., & Lee, Y. (1998). Joint modeling of mean and dispersion. *Technometrics, 40*(2), 168–171.

Nelder, J. A., & Lee, Y. (2002). Likelihood Quasi-likelihood and pseudolikelihood: Some comparisons. *Journal of the Royal Statistical Society: Series B. Methodological, 54*(1), 273–284.

Nelder, J. A., & Wedderburn, R. W. M. (1972). Generalized linear models. *Journal of the Royal Statistical Society: Series A. General, 135*(3), 370–384.

Paul, S. R., & Islam, A. S. (1998). Joint estimation of the mean and dispersion parameters in the analysis of proportions: A comparison of efficiency and bias. *The Canadian Journal of Statistics, 26*(1), 83–94.

Pregibon, D. (1984). Generalized linear models: Book review. *The Annals of Statistics, 12*(4), 1589–1596.

Smyth, G. K. (1989). Generalized linear models with varying dispersion. *Journal of the Royal Statistical Society: Series B. Methodological, 51*(1), 47–60.

Smyth, G. K., & Verbyla, A. P. (1999). Adjusted likelihood methods for modelling dispersion in generalized linear models. *Environmetrics, 10*(6), 695–709.

Wu, L., & Li, H. (2012). Variable selection for joint mean and dispersion models of the inverse Gaussian distribution. *Metrika, 75*(6), 795–808.

Part V
Case Studies- USA Election 2020 and Netherlands COVID

Chapter 13
Case Studies: Election Data and COVID Data

13.1 Two Case Studies- Election and COVID

In this chapter, we use models introduced throughout other chapters in this book to analyze hypotheses related to two different cases. One example is based on data obtained at a single point in time, and the other is based on data collected over time from several respondents. In particular, we examined two case studies, *Election data* in United States of America and *COVID data* obtained in the Netherlands.

The election data analysis can be used as a guided process that demonstrates how statistical models are used to identify key information that the data reveal, while the *COVID data* provides an opportunity for the reader to explore possible questions that can be addressed as data are collected on an ongoing basis.

13.2 USA 2020 Election Data

13.2.1 Election Data Questions

Imagine you are the campaign manager for one of the two major parties and you learned that you have access to the results of 2020 US presidential data by counties and states as you prepare for 2024 presidential elections. What questions would you want to ask of the data? A set of possible questions may be:

1. What are the key county factors that impacted the outcome of the election?
2. How did my candidate perform in votes across the 12 swing states?
3. What messaging resonated most with voters, and what messaging fell flat?
4. What were the most significant policy issues driving voter turnout, and how can we better align our platform with voter priorities in 2024?

J. R. Wilson et al., *Modeling Binary Correlated Responses*, ICSA Book Series in Statistics, https://doi.org/10.1007/978-3-031-62427-8_13

5. How did external factors such as the COVID-19 pandemic, economic conditions, and social unrest affect voter sentiment and hence their vote.

13.2.2 Election Variables and Data Analysis

We examined the 2020 presidential election data based on what was made available. For this discussion, we selected 12 states that were matched for location and population. There are six states that voted for the Democratic candidate [Arizona, California, Georgia, Illinois, New York, and Pennsylvania] and six states that voted for the Republican candidate [Florida, Indiana, Ohio, Texas, South Carolina, and Utah]. Votes for each candidate by state and county were summed and compared using a binary outcome variable (0 = Democratic candidate won state/county; 1 = Republican candidate won state/county). The data are given by county and state.

https://dataverse.harvard.edu/dataset.xhtml?persistentId=doi:10.7910/DVN/42MVDX. In addition, we had the socioeconomic factors as well as poverty estimates from the US Department of Commerce, Bureau of the Census, Small Area Income and Poverty Estimates (SAIPE) Program (https://www.census.gov/programs-surveys/saipe.html). The data contained the following summary values and presented by counties within states and type of county: metro counties, non-metro counties, and estimate of people of all ages in poverty 2021. A subset of these data is given in the Table 13.1.

We used the logistic regression model as presented in Chap. 3, where vote is the binary response with 1 denoting the county voted as a majority for the Republican candidate and 0 was for the Democratic candidate. The logistic regression method can be used to predict the probability of a county voting for a Republican candidate

Table 13.1 Election results for some counties

State	County	Vote	Number in poverty	Median household income
AZ	Arizona	0	919,680	68,967
AZ	Apache County	0	18,422	41,002
AZ	Cochise County	1	20,618	55,748
AZ	Coconino County	0	22,677	63,829
AZ	Maricopa County	0	502,224	76,230
AZ	Yavapai County	1	29,766	57,676
AZ	Yuma County	1	34,270	55,991
FL	Florida	1	2,830,813	63,054
FL	Alachua County	0	50,668	56,006
FL	Baker County	1	4187	60,994
FL	Bay County	1	24,383	60,106
FL	Bradford County	1	4636	54,911
FL	Brevard County	1	68,879	65,280
FL	Duval County	0	146,090	60,121

based on various predictor variables, such as demographic characteristics, socioeconomic factors, political affiliation, etc. A logistic regression analysis can determine which predictor variables have a significant impact on the likelihood of voting for one candidate over another. The model helps identify key factors influencing voting behavior. The logistic regression model can be evaluated to assess its overall fit and predictive performance. This involves examining measures such as model accuracy, the area under the receiver operating characteristic (ROC) curve, and Hosmer-Lemeshow goodness-of-fit test. Moreover, logistic regression allows for the interpretation of the direction and strength of relationships between predictor variables and the likelihood of a county voting for a candidate. This helps understand the underlying dynamics driving voting behavior. As we discussed in Chap. 3, logistic regression assumes certain conditions, such as linearity of the logit and independence of observations, and these assumptions can be evaluated using diagnostic tests to ensure the validity of the model results. However, if the necessary predictors do not exist to address the questions, then we will outline the added additional information or methodology needed.

As we examined the election data, one wonders if logistic regression in Chap. 3 is the most appropriate as the results in a county nested within a state are not generated based on independent trials. Maybe, the methods in Chap. 9 are better suited where counties are nested within states, where states can be seen as a random effect.

We fit a model with the covariates as given and the county's majority voting preferences. The overall impact of these covariates in voting by county is measured based on its p-value. Those with $p < 0.05$ are considered significant, and those with $p < 0.0001$ are considered extremely significant. We present the results in Table 13.2 with states is a fixed effect.

We fit a random effects model where we treated the 12 states as a sample of the population of 50 states. Treating states as random effect showed that it was the correct decision since the variance among states was estimated to be larger than 1.96.

Table 13.2 Parameter estimates in voting preferences at swing states (Utah is reference state)

Parameter	Estimate	Standard error	p-value
AZ	−0.9453	0.5068	0.0622
CA	−1.5584	0.2788	<0.0001
FL	0.0485	0.3223	0.8804
GA	−0.2654	0.2194	0.2263
IL	0.2812	0.2831	0.3206
IN	1.3456	0.4352	0.0020
NY	−0.7055	0.2736	0.0099
OH	1.0012	0.3848	0.0093
PA	−0.1129	0.3013	0.7080
SC	−0.7648	0.3261	0.0190
TX	0.7796	0.2366	0.0010
Number in poverty	−1.99E-6	6.062E-7	0.0010
Median household income	−0.00002	5.705E-6	0.0003

Table 13.3 State are seen as a sample of the 50 states

Subject	Estimate	Std err pred	p-value
State AZ	−0.6247	0.4930	0.2054
State CA	−1.3765	0.3470	<0.0001
State FL	0.06016	0.3744	0.8724
State GA	−0.2296	0.3112	0.4609
State IL	0.2680	0.3488	0.4425
State IN	1.0589	0.4133	0.0105
State NY	−0.6130	0.3462	0.0769
State OH	0.8279	0.3975	0.0375
State PA	−0.08022	0.3625	0.8249
State SC	−0.6323	0.3815	0.0978
State TX	0.7408	0.3187	0.0203
State UT	0.6006	0.4861	0.2169

However, the states showed variation in their values, Table 13.3. There is definitely significant variation in the states of California, Indiana, Ohio, and Texas.

13.2.3 Election Data Interpretation

Let us revisit the questions and what can we address.

1. What are the key county factors that impacted the outcome of the election?

   Response: We found from Table 13.2 that *number in poverty* ($p < 0.0001$) and *median household income* ($p < 0.002$) are key factors in winning the county elections. We found counties with higher numbers in poverty were more likely to vote democrats and those with lower median household income were more likely to vote for the democrats.
2. How do these results differ across the 12 swing states on average?

   Response: We found from Table 13.3 that CA, IL, PA, and NY preferred the Democratic candidate while Texas and Florida preferred the Republican candidate.
   For questions 3, 4, and 5, while they are noteworthy, the data were not available to answer. In questions:
3. What messaging resonated most with voters, and what messaging fell flat?
4. What were the most significant policy issues driving voter turnout, and how can we better align our platform with voter priorities?

   Response: To answer such questions and determine how the results differ among characteristics about voters, we would need to have exit surveys to have that data determine the impact. If we were to measure that information as a binary response, then we can use a logistic regression model and obtain the odds.

However, if we do those outcomes on a continuous measure, we can use regression analysis, which was not covered in this book but can be seen in Wilson et al. (2023).

5. How did external factors such as the COVID-19 pandemic, economic conditions, and social unrest affect voter sentiment and hence their vote.

   Response: We can obtain voters opinion on the handling of COVID-19 pandemic, economic conditions, and social unrest on some scale. They can be binary or ordered or some linear range of scores and their vote as the response, and one can use a logistic regression model to answer how these issues affected the vote. In the event that one shares the belief that counties are nested within states, then a logistic regression model with random effects is fitted, Table 13.3.

13.3 The Netherlands 2020–2021 COVID Data

In the analysis of these COVID data, we treated them as case-control studies, although the data were originally collected prospectively. This is indeed a valuable research strategy, especially when investigating rare events and exploring potential determinants or risk factors. Case-control studies are particularly useful when studying rare outcomes or events because researchers can intentionally oversample cases (individuals exhibiting the phenomenon of interest) to ensure an adequate sample size for analysis (Fang et al., 2015).

In these COVID data, we have 4725 deceased cases and 2,062,936 non-deceased cases. To conduct a binary model of any kind using all the data will not be an optimal use of statistical methods. The ratio of deceased to non-deceased is about 434 to 1. Thus, deceased cases are rare. We took a matched sample of cases to control in the ratio of 1 to 10. While we focus on model fitting, it is also helpful to mention that case-control designs are often more efficient than other study designs, such as cohort studies, because they allow researchers to focus resources and efforts on identifying and recruiting cases while selecting controls from the same source population. By comparing cases and controls, researchers can identify differences in potential determinants or risk factors associated with the occurrence of the COVID disease. It helps elucidate the underlying causes. Case-control designs are well-suited for studying binary outcomes, where observations either exhibit the phenomenon of interest (cases) or do not (controls). This simplicity in outcome measurement facilitates analysis and interpretation. Also, when rigorously conducted, case-control studies can provide robust evidence to support or refute hypotheses about the determinants of a given phenomenon. This can enhance confidence in research findings and contribute to evidence-based decision-making.

Dr. Marcus *writes* "The Dutch government tries hard to provide open data, although what is provided only scratches the surface due to GDPR. Its biggest dataset contains around 2 million observations of people tested positive, their age, sex, the province where they were tested, and if they had to be admitted to the hospital and/or died." We use these data as a means of providing the reader with an example but knowing that these data have several limitations. Also, we use a sample of these observations.

13.3.1 COVID Data Questions

A list of questions emanated from the very thought that data in regard to COVID was available in another form in another country. By addressing these questions and conducting a rigorous analysis of the clustered COVID-19 mortality and hospitalization data using logistic regression, one can gain valuable insights into the factors influencing outcomes and inform evidence-based strategies for managing the next pandemic. Our access to COVID data in the Netherlands covers the period 2021–2022 and was limited in scope. However, an analysis of the COVID data allows the reader to explore and practice analyzing and reporting techniques found within earlier chapters. Here are some possible questions a researcher knowing that COVID data were available may want to ask even before he/she sees the data.

1. Do age, gender, and quarter in the Netherlands impact the death rate?
2. Given the data situation, what are the odds that a man died in quarter 1 as opposed to a woman?
3. How do the mortality rates among different provinces compare?
4. Are there any emerging variants of the virus that might be contributing to changes in mortality rates, and if so, what are their characteristics and implications?
5. How can public health messaging and policies be adjusted to better address the factors contributing to COVID-19 mortality and mitigate its effects?

These questions reflect the unique role of physicians in providing direct patient care, counseling, and support during the COVID-19 pandemic.

Inspired by the article by Dr. Marc Jacobs, we examined clustered data from provinces in the Netherlands about the probabilities of death after 30 days when tested positive. Hospitalizations and mortality due to COVID-19 across a one-year span is listed. (https://medium.com/@marc.jacobs012/predicting-covid-19-mortality-using-logistic-regression-in-sas-5453d3532cd7) (*Data source*: https://data.rivm.nl/covid-19/).

13.3.2 COVID Data Variables and Analysis

A subset of these data is given in Table 13.4. These are 11 of more than 2 million cases represented. For each case, we have gender (male or female), the quarter (one of 4 quarters), the age group (10 age groups 0–9; 10–19; 20–29; 30–39; 40–49; 50–59; 60–69; 70–79; 80–89; 90+), and the 12 provinces.

Table 13.4 A subset of COVID data

Obs	Deceased	Sex	Quarter	Age	Province
2	No	Female	1	0	Utrecht
3	No	Male	1	0	Drenthe
4	No	Male	1	0	Utrecht
5	No	Female	1	0	FryslÃ¢n
6	No	Male	1	0	Groningen
7	No	Male	1	0	Drenthe
8	No	Female	1	0	Limburg
9	No	Male	1	0	Gelderland
10	No	Male	1	0	Noord-Holland
11	No	Male	1	0	Gelderland
12	No	Female	1	0	Noord-Holland

13.3.3 COVID Data Interpretation

The results show that men were 1.72 times more likely to be deceased. Older folks were more likely to be deceased. One was more likely to be deceased in Q1 as opposed to Q4 but less likely to be deceased than in Q4. Not being familiar with the area and rather going purely on the results, we used Zuid-Holland as our yardstick. On average, dying from COVID was about the same for most provinces when compared to Zuid-Holland. However, FryslÃ¢n, Gelderland, Overijssel, and Utrecht were significantly different in death rates as opposed to Zuid-Holland. More deadly than Zuid-Holland were Gelderland and Utrecht.

Let us revisit the questions and what can we address.

1. Do age, gender, and quarter in the Netherlands impact the death rate?

   Response: Yes, we found from Table 13.5 that age gender and the quarter had an impact on the mortality rate.
2. Given the data situation, what are the odds that a man died in quarter 1 as opposed to a woman?

   Response: Men were 1.72 times more likely to die than women.
3. How do the mortality rates among different provinces compare?

   Response: One was more likely to die in the Gelderland and Utrecht provinces.
4. Are there any emerging variants of the virus that might be contributing to changes in mortality rates, and if so, what are their characteristics and implications?

   Response: As for question 4, we do not have the data to answer that question. If we had environmental measures or some way to measure the variants, then yes, we can address the question.
5. How can public health messaging and policies be adjusted to better address the factors contributing to COVID-19 mortality and mitigate its effects?

Table 13.5 Covariates impact on death

Parameter	Estimate	Standard error	p-value	Odds
Female	−0.2711	0.0210	<0.0001	0.581
Age	0.1375	0.00189	<0.0001	1.147
Q1	0.3000	0.0453	<0.0001	0.956
Q2	−0.00534	0.0675	0.9370	0.704
Q3	−0.6400	0.0611	<0.0001	0.373
Drenthe	0.2593	0.1329	0.0509	1.076
Flevoland	−0.0411	0.1358	0.7621	0.797
FryslÃ¢n	−0.2369	0.1115	0.0337	0.655
Gelderland	0.1799	0.0542	0.0009	0.994
Groningen	−0.2210	0.1232	0.0729	0.666
Limburg	0.0518	0.0650	0.4260	0.875
Noord-Brabant	0.0633	0.0592	0.2852	0.885
Noord-Holland	−0.0390	0.0537	0.4684	0.799
Overijssel	−0.3543	0.0771	<0.0001	0.583
Utrecht	0.2476	0.0848	0.0035	1.064
Zeeland	−0.0953	0.1162	0.4122	0.755

These questions reflect the unique role of physicians in providing direct patient care, counseling, and support during the COVID-19 pandemic. Public awareness and the communication with the public on health issues are important measures to have to address such a question.

References

Fang, D., Chong, J., & Wilson, J. R. (2015). Predicted probabilities' relationship to inclusion probabilities. *American Journal of Public Health, 105*(5), 837–839.

Wilson, J., Chen, D.-G., & Peace, K. E. (2023). *Statistical analytics for health data science with SAS and R* (1st ed.). Chapman and Hall/CRC.

Index

J. R. Wilson et al., *Modeling Binary Correlated Responses*, ICSA Book Series in Statistics, https://doi.org/10.1007/978-3-031-62427-8

Printed by Printforce, the Netherlands